SO-ANG-284

Treatment of Sex Offenders in Social Work and Mental Health Settings

The *Journal of Social Work & Human Sexuality* series:

- *Social Work and Child Sexual Abuse*, edited by Jon R. Conte and David A. Shore

- *Human Sexuality in Medical Social Work*, edited by Larry Lister and David A. Shore

- *Homosexuality and Social Work*, edited by Robert Schoenberg and Richard Goldberg, with David A. Shore

- *Feminist Perspectives on Social Work and Human Sexuality*, edited by Mary Valentich and James Gripton

- *Social Work Practice in Sexual Problems*, edited by James Gripton and Mary Valentich

- *Human Sexuality, Ethnoculture and Social Work*, edited by Larry Lister

- *Adolescent Sexualities: Overviews and Principles of Intervention*, edited by Paula Allen-Meares and David A. Shore

- *Intimate Relationships: Some Social Work Perspectives on Love*, edited by Wendell Ricketts and Harvey L. Gochros

- *Infertility and Adoption: A Guide for Social Work Practice*, edited by Deborah Valentine

- *Sociopsychological Aspects of Sexually Transmitted Diseases*, edited by Margaret Rodway and Marianne Wright

- *The Sexually Unusual: Guide to Understanding and Helping*, edited by Dennis M. Dailey

- *Treatment of Sex Offenders in Social Work and Mental Health Settings*, edited by John S. Wodarski and Daniel L. Whitaker

Treatment of Sex Offenders in Social Work and Mental Health Settings

John S. Wodarski
Daniel L. Whitaker
Editors

The Haworth Press
New York • London

Treatment of Sex Offenders in Social Work and Mental Health Settings has also been published as *Journal of Social Work & Human Sexuality*, Volume 7, Number 2 1988.

The Haworth Press, Inc., 12 West 32 Street, New York, NY 10001
EUROSPAN/Haworth, 3 Henrietta Street, London WC2E 8LU England

LIBRARY OF CONGRESS
Library of Congress Cataloging-in-Publication Data

Treatment of sex offenders in social work and mental health settings / John S. Wodarski, Daniel L. Whitaker, editors.
    p. cm.
    "Has also been published as Journal of social work & human sexuality, volume 7, number 2, 1988" – T.p. verso.
    Includes bibliographies and index.
    ISBM 0-86656-791-7
    1. Sex offenders – Rehabilitation – United States. 2. Community mental health services – United States. 3. Family psychotherapy – United States. 4. Family social work – United States. 5. Sex offenders – United States – Family relationships. I. Wodarski, John S. II. Whitaker, Daniel L.
    [DNLM: 1. Community Mental Health Services. 2. Sex Offenses. W1JO889D v. 7 / WM 610 T7835]
HQ72.U53T74   1988
365'.66 – dc19
DNLM/DLC
for Library of Congress   88-16422
                                                            CIP

Treatment of Sex Offenders in Social Work and Mental Health Settings

CONTENTS

ABOUT THE EDITORS

John S. Wodarski, PhD, is Professor of Social Work and Director of the Research Center at The University of Georgia School of Social Work. He has held research and teaching positions at Washington University School of Social Work in St. Louis, Missouri; The Institute for Behavioral Research, Inc., in Silver Spring, Maryland; The Johns Hopkins University Center for Social Organization of Schools in Baltimore, Maryland; and The University of Maryland School of Social Work and Community Planning in Baltimore, Maryland.

Daniel L. Whitaker, MSW, is Research Associate in the field of the treatment of addictive behaviors at the University of Washington Center for Social Welfare Research in Seattle, Washington. Previously, he was Senior Therapist of the North Cobb Community Mental Health Center's Sex Offender Treatment Program in Atlanta, Georgia.

Contributors

John M. Achterkirchen, MSW, Psychiatric Social Worker, Sex Offender Treatment and Evaluation Project, Department of Mental Health, Atascadero State Hospital, Atascadero, California.

Peggy Cleveland, PhD, Assistant Professor, School of Social Work, University of Georgia, Athens, Georgia.

Diana J. English, PhD, Division of Children and Family Services, Department of Social and Health Services, Olympia, Washington.

John E. Henderson, MSW, Division of Children's and Family Services, Department of Social and Health Services, Everett, Washington.

Lettie L. Lockhart, PhD, Assistant Professor, School of Social Work, University of Georgia, Athens, Georgia.

Ward R. MacKenzie, MSW, Child Protective Services Caseworker, Coordinator, Eastside Mental Health Juvenile Sexual Offender Treatment Program, Division of Children's and Family Services, Department of Social and Health Services, Everett, Washington.

Janice Marques, PhD, Sex Offender Treatment and Evaluation Project, Department of Mental Health, Atascadero State Hospital, Atascadero, California.

Michael H. Miner, PhD, Experimental Psychologist, Sex Offender Treatment and Evaluation Project, Department of Mental Health, Atascadero State Hospital, Atascadero, California.

Craig Nelson, PhD, Sex Offender Treatment and Evaluation Project, Department of Mental Health, Atascadero State Hospital, Atascadero, California.

Louise Prince, Sociology Department, University of California, Riverside, California.

Kabe Russell, MSW, LCSW, Sex Offender Treatment and Evaluation Project, Department of Mental Health, Atascadero State Hospital, Atascadero, California.

Inger J. Sagatun, PhD, Associate Professor, Administration of Justice Department, School of Applied Arts and Sciences, San Jose State University, San Jose, California.

Benjamin E. Saunders, PhD, Assistant Professor, Director, Child Assault Program, Crime Victims Research and Treatment Center, Department of Psychiatry and Behavioral Sciences, Medical University of South Carolina, Charleston, South Carolina.

Robert F. Schilling, PhD, Assistant Professor, School of Social Work, Columbia University, New York, New York.

Steven P. Schinke, PhD, Professor, School of Social Work, Columbia University, New York, New York.

Linda G. Tosti-Lane, Division of Children and Family Services, Department of Social and Health Services, Mountlake Terrace, Washington.

Daniel L. Whitaker, MSW, Research Associate, Center for Social Welfare Research, University of Washington, Seattle, Washington.

John S. Wodarski, PhD, Professor, Director, Research Center, School of Social Work, University of Georgia, Athens, Georgia.

Preface

The focus of this text is on social work practice with sexual offenders in community mental health settings. The sexual offender is being turned away in many cases from psychiatric hospitals and is being served in open community centers. Due to the significant increase in the number of clients served, professionals in mental health centers and related human service agencies must be equipped to deal with the offender with valid, up-to-date information.

The nature of the chapters cover three major classifications: the incest offender, the violent offender, and the social decency offender. The text is of particular interest to psychiatrists, psychologists, social workers, and other professionals in mental health settings.

The chapters consist of theoretical and empirical data to substantiate the practice principles derived. The articles provide social workers practicing in mental health settings with up-to-date theoretical issues, an evaluation of the empirical base, and practice principles derived from the theoretical and empirical base.

The article by Lockhart, Saunders, and Cleveland, entitled "Adult Male Sexual Offenders: An Overview of Treatment Techniques," elucidates the variety of approaches that are available for treating sex offenders in social work and mental health settings. The authors do an exquisite job of evaluating the treatment approaches, elucidating issues in the area, and specifying what approaches are appropriate.

The next article, entitled "Mentally Retarded Sex Offenders: Fact, Fiction, and Treatment," by Schilling and Schinke presents a penetrating review of the basic issue regarding sexual offenders and mental retardation. This nonbiased review elucidates the data base and future research questions that need to be addressed.

The article entitled "Treatment of Sexual Offenders in a Community Mental Health Center: An Evaluation" by Whitaker and

Wodarski elucidates criteria for determining whether sexual deviants are dangerous, outlines procedures for evaluating treatment, and provides an example of how single case designs can be utilized in a community mental health center to evaluate a comprehensive treatment program based on the social skills model. The article also elucidates the use of multimeasurement and the complexity of evaluating behavioral change.

Next, the article entitled "Incest Family Dynamics: Family Members' Perceptions Before and After Therapy" by Sagatun and Prince relates how perceptions of perpetrators and abusers affect how they view each other and has implications for treatment.

The article entitled "Family Centered Casework Practice with Sexually Aggressive Children" by Henderson, English, and MacKenzie is a fascinating article in its elaboration of beginning knowledge in the field. It employs empirical methodologies such as the development of a risk assessment scale necessary to identify sexually aggressive children. The authors provide an excellent example of pilot research executed by social work practitioners.

The article entitled "Child Protective Service Workers' Ratings of Likely Emotional Trauma to Child Sexual Abuse Victims" by English and Tosti-Lane is another outstanding contribution that elucidates the incidence of sexual assault among adolescents and sexual assault among children toward children. How professionals view differently the various types of child abuse is discussed, and implications are drawn.

The article "Relapse Prevention: A Cognitive-Behavioral Model for Treatment of the Rapist and Child Molester" by Nelson et al. provides a critical analysis of child molestation and the rapist. The authors present a comprehensive intervention program that is based on theory and research.

The final article by Wodarski and Whitaker, entitled "Issues in Treating Sex Offenders in the Community," suggests issues requiring resolution to facilitate the effective treatment of sexual offenders in social work and mental health settings.

John S. Wodarski

Adult Male Sexual Offenders:
An Overview of Treatment Techniques

Lettie L. Lockhart
Benjamin E. Saunders
Peggy Cleveland

SUMMARY. A review of common treatment approaches used with adult sex offenders was presented. Treatment approaches reviewed included: psychodynamic, behavioral, cognitive, skills educational training, family-system, pharmacological, and surgical therapies. While many procedures have some empirical and clinical support, claims regarding treatment effectiveness must be carefully scrutinized in view of the difficulties of formulating and operationalizing criteria for effectiveness, the lack of rigorous empirical evaluation of most therapies, and the lack of long-term follow-up. Future research should focus on the following: (1) The extension and refinement of assessment methods that will serve to discriminate sex offenders from other persons and different types of sex offenders from each other; (2) future development of, and rigorous comparison among, treatment techniques effectiveness; and (3) long-term follow-up of sexual offenders who have been treated with different methods.

Over the past two decades there has been a growing awareness of the high prevalence of sexual aggression and sexual victimization in our culture. Appropriately, the initial focus of most sexual assault research and treatment was on the severe consequences suffered by victims (Veronen & Kilpatrick, 1980; Burgess & Holmstrom, 1974; Albin, 1977). Sexual offenders were viewed with moral outrage, disgust, and anger; and long periods of incarceration or even death were seen as justified societal reactions. Realistically, three alternatives have been available to the criminal justice system for dealing with apprehended sexual offenders: (1) determinate incarceration in correctional facilities; (2) indeterminate incarceration in state mental health institutions; or (3) court-ordered probation, sometimes

© 1989 by The Haworth Press, Inc. All rights reserved. *1*

coupled with various forms of treatment (Clark, 1986; Freeman-Longo, 1986; Freeman-Longo & Wall, 1986). Numerous studies have documented that a strictly punitive approach to managing sexual offenders is prohibitively expensive, is implemented relatively infrequently, and simply does not prevent reoffenses (McCahill, Meyer, & Fischman, 1979; Grunfeld and Noreik, 1986; West, Roy, & Nichols, 1978).

Community victimization and offender studies have demonstrated that only a small percentage of offenders are ever apprehended and that even those rarely serve long prison terms (Kilpatrick, Veronen, Saunders, Best, Amick-McMullan, & Paduhovich, 1987; Abel, Becker, Mittleman, Cunningham-Rathner, Roulean, & Murphy, 1987; Knopp, 1984). In many cases, imprisonment, far from being a deterrent to reoffending, exacerbates offenders' tendency and ability to commit sexual assaults. Freeman-Longo and Wall (1986) suggested that breaking the chain of sexual aggression requires not only imprisonment but also effective treatment. The purpose of this article is to review the literature on the treatment of sexual offenders, describe several treatment approaches that have been used with this population, and make recommendations for future clinical research. The review is limited to the treatment of adult male offenders who commit one or more types of sexual assault against adults or children of either gender. In this paper, sexual assaults are categorized as rape, molestation, or noncontact assaults. Rape is defined as the actual or attempted penetration of the vagina, anus, or mouth by the penis, finger, or an object, using force or the threat of force. Molestation is defined as physical sexual contact that does not include penetration, using force or threat of force. Noncontact assaults include sexual offenses that do not involve actual physical contact, such as exhibitionism and voyeurism.

INCIDENCE AND PREVALENCE

In 1985, the Federal Bureau of Investigation reported that 87,340 forcible rapes perpetrated against females were reported to the police (FBI, 1986). However, victimization surveys of community samples indicate that reported offenses represent only a fraction of the sexual assaults that actually occur. For example, Kilpatrick, Veronen, Saunders, Best, Amick-McMullan, and Paduhovich (1987) reported that fewer than 7% of the child or adult sexual assaults committed against their community sample of 391 women were ever reported to the police. Therefore, the true annual incidence of sexual assault is likely to be from two to twenty times greater than the assaults reported to authorities depending upon the type of offense. Current lifetime prevalence estimates suggest that 50% of all women and 15% of men will be victims of a form of sexual assault at some time in their lives (Johnson, 1980; Silberman, 1980; Ageton, 1983; Peters, Wyatt, & Finkelhor, 1986; Russell, 1984; Koss, Gidycz, & Wisniewski, 1987; Kilpatrick, Best, Veronen, Amick, Villeponteaux, & Ruff, 1985; Kilpatrick, Saunders, Veronen, Best, & Von, 1987; Saunders, Villeponteaux, Kilpatrick, & Veronen, 1987).

Estimates of the number of men who commit sexual offenses or the number of offenses they commit are more difficult to develop since only a very small proportion are ever arrested and convicted (Clark & Lewis, 1977). Rapaport and Burkhart (1984) found that 15% of their sample of college men admitted to obtaining sexual intercourse against the wills of their female dates. In a national sample of 2,972 college men, Koss, Gidycz, and Wisniewski (1987) found that in the previous six month period prior to the survey, 7.7% of the respondents reported perpetrating at least one act that met legal definitions of rape and that virtually none had come in contact with the criminal justice system. In a previous set of studies, Koss and colleagues (Koss & Oros, 1982; Koss, 1985; Koss, Leonard, Beezley, & Oros, 1985) found that 4.6% of a sample of 1,846 college males acknowledged committing acts that met legal definitions of rape. Able, Becker, Mittleman, Cunningham-Rathner, Rouleau, and Murphy (1987) reported on the types and number of offenses committed by a sample of 561 sex offenders in outpatient treatment. They reported that these offenders had committed an average of 2.02 paraphiliac acts. The average number of acts committed and victims assaulted varied widely by paraphilia. For example, the average rapist had committed 7.2 rapes against 7.0 victims, and child molesters with nonfamilial male victims committed an average of 281.7 assaults against 150.2 victims. Abel, Becker, Cunningham-Rathner, Rouleau, Kaplan, and Reich (1984) estimated very conservatively that only 1 in 60 sexual crimes actually leads to arrest. Together these studies indicate that adult male sexual aggression and subsequent sexual victimization are serious social problems that affect a large portion of the population.

TREATMENT APPROACHES

Although significant differences exist in the theories of etiology and change on which different treatment approaches are based, there is common agreement that a substantial number of sex offenders begin their sexually assaultive behavior as adolescents, that sexual offenders develop patterns of assaultive behavior that are chronic and habitual, and that the earlier intervention begins, the greater the potential for disrupting these patterns of behavior (Knopp, 1984; Becker, Cunningham-Rathner, & Kaplan, 1986). Many experts have noted the similarities between sex offenders and persons with other addictive patterns of behavior such as substance abuse (Dreiblatt, 1982; Laws, 1980). The goal of most treatment approaches is to teach sexual offenders how to recognize, acknowledge, and control their sexually abusive or assaultive behavior. This goal implies that good candidates for treatment must have a strong motivation to end their deviant sexual behavior and have the cognitive ability to learn new skills. Most treatment programs have thorough assessment components designed to select appropriate candidates and employ a variety of treatment techniques. Veterans in the area of sex offender treatment eschew the word "cure," for no one claims that treatment approaches and programs will end the problems. Readers are cautioned to keep this in mind as they read the following section on the various treatment approaches.

Psychodynamic Approaches

Individual and Group Psychotherapy

The pioneer sex-offender treatment programs were based primarily on the traditional medical or psychiatric model. The preferred forms of treatment were individual psychotherapy and concomitant group psychotherapy, both usually conducted by a male therapist. Psychoanalytic and other psychodynamic theories were the primary perspectives used for treating sexual offenders prior to the 1960s. Karpman (1954) and Lorand and Balint (1956) provide an intensive review of these early treatment approaches. Individual therapy typically addressed the interplay of intrapsychic and personality dynamics and the resulting intrapersonal conflicts. These were assumed to account for both the etiology of the problem and its change during treatment (Kopp, 1962; Riemann, 1968; Crown, 1983). Group therapy was based on interactional theory and group dynamics (Hartman, 1965; Quinsey, 1977; Resink & Peters, 1967; Peters, Pedigo, Steg, & McKenna, 1968; Roether & Peters, 1972; Hobbs, 1980). The focus of treatment was on personal growth and the resolution of intrapersonal conflicts through the development of personal insight.

There is little systemic empirical information available to provide the basis for making decisions as to the usefulness of these approaches to the treatment of sex offenders. Romero and Williams (1983) reported on a 10-year longitudinal experimental study of sex offenders participating in a program of intensive probation supervision and group psychotherapy or probation alone. Using recidivism as the basis for evaluation of the long-term effects of the program, they concluded that group psychotherapy in addition to probation supervision does not significantly reduce sex offense recidivism when compared to intensive probation supervision alone. However, they cautioned against relying solely on these findings in making policy decisions about the continuation or termination of group psychotherapy due to methodological problems in their investigation (e.g., use of recidivism as sole outcome measure of the effectiveness of intervention, use of arrest data only, and small sample size to detect significant differences).

Fantasy-Oriented Psychotherapy

Matek (1985-86) stated that many sex offenders can be helped by making use of fantasy training as an additional approach to traditional psychotherapy. He suggested that action-prone aggressive, impulsive, socially deviant, nonpsychotic individuals generally lack skills in the use of fantasy. Ferenczi (1926) recommended that fantasy-oriented psychotherapy should be used only at the end of a psychoanalysis, and that it be limited to three major themes; sexuality, specifically masturbation fantasies; infancy related fantasies; and fantasies associated with psychoanalytic transference. Cohn (1966) stated:

> Fantasies consist of bits and pieces of memories, thoughts, images, and sound. They are a sequence of associations organized into various forms and shapes. They have personal meanings . . . they arise on the triple-track of sensations, emotions and intellect. (p. 221)

Gebhard, Gagon, Pomeroy, and Christenson (1965) found many differences in the fantasy activities of different groups of sexual offenders. Rapists showed the lowest level of fantasy activity, and pedophiles engaged in the most. They concluded that after working with masturbatory fantasies of pedophiles fantasy therapy may be useful, but the use of this intervention with sexual aggressives such as rapists would be much more complicated. Groth (1979) explained that traditional psychotherapy is not effective with most rapists because, "It requires traits not usually found in rapists: self-observation, intelligence, capacity for abstract thinking, motivation for change, persistence, and the ability to endure discomfort" (p. 216). Spanos (1971) suggested that fantasy is a precursor to behavior and that constructive alternative behavior responses can be added to a person's behavior repertoire by incorporating them into their fantasies (Abel & Blanchard, 1974).

Hypnotic Uncovering Techniques

Stava (1984) conducted a single subject study to determine whether hypnotic uncovering techniques can be effective in reducing inappropriate sexual excitation in pedophilia. The primary hypnotic uncovering techniques used in his study were induced dreams, described by Sacerdote (1967), and the affect bridge technique, described by Watkins (1971). In Stava's examination of the literature, he was able to locate only one brief case study conducted by Caprio (1972); but the treatment techniques were unclear, and measures of treatment outcome were lacking. In addition, he concluded that recent treatment approaches of sexual offenders have primarily used behavioral interventions (Foote & Laws, 1981; Josiassen, Fantuzzo, & Rosen, 1980; Laws, 1980; Quinsey, Chaplin, & Carrigan, 1980; Wong, Gaydos, & Fuqua, 1982; Kilmann, Sabalis, Gearing, Bukstel, & Scovern, 1982). In contrast, Stava used hypnotic techniques within a psychodynamic framework and several objective measures of penile tumescence to measure treatment effects. Hypnotherapy consisted of 25 sessions over a period of approximately 9 months. These sessions began with a hypnotic induction and a variety of deepening techniques until adequate trance depth was obtained. At that point, it was suggested that the patient would experience a hypnotic dream that was either directly or indirectly related to his sexual problems. The patient would report the dream as it occurred. Rather than having the patient to retroactively associate the dream after its occurrence, he was instructed instead to dream additional dreams which were suggested to be related to the original dream (Sacerdote, 1967).

The affect bridge technique (Watkins, 1971) was used with the hypnotic technique. This technique involves suggesting that the patient allow an affect that he is currently experiencing to carry him back in time to a situation in the past when he was experiencing a similar emotion. At the end of treatment, Stava (1984) reported that psychophysiological measures revealed a definite reduction of sexual excitation to slides of prepubescent children. He concluded that the psychodynamic hypnotherapeutic approach to male pedophilia appears to be effective. It is suggested that the uncovering of repressed traumatic materials, the reliving of emotionally laden experiences, and the experience of pleasurable fantasies of appropriate behavior in a safe therapeutic environment may have been involved in producing the treatment effects.

Recent Developments

The early sex offender treatment programs were, to a large degree, captive to the prevailing idea that sex offenders were generally unfulfilled men, suffering from extreme intrapsychic conflicts and carried away by sudden, uncontrollable surges of sexual desire

(Knopp, 1984), and that insight-oriented therapy could relieve these conflicts and change the behavior. Two factors greatly affected the direction of sex-offender treatment. The first was the gradual move away from this "medical," psychiatric, or intrapsychic conflict model of treatment to an approach that focuses on the deviant behavior itself. Traditional psychodynamically-based approaches have proved unsatisfactory in stopping the violent behavior and are very expensive to deliver (Knopp, 1976, pp. 138-139). Also, as the prevalence of sexual aggression has become better understood and professionals have had more experience with nonincarcerated offenders who are generally more functional, it has become clear that only a relatively small proportion of these men suffer from diagnosable psychiatric disorders (Saunders, McClure, & Murphy, 1986). Therefore, programs aimed at diagnosing psychiatric disorders, promoting personal growth, or resolving intrapersonal conflicts through psychodynamic therapy have become the exception rather than the rule (Knopp, 1984; Quinsey, 1977).

A second factor influencing traditional psychodynamic views of sexual deviancy has been the impact of feminist theory on our understanding of sexual aggression (Brownmiller, 1975; Russell, 1975; Knopp, 1984; Clark, 1986). Feminist theory has described the cultural and sex role attitudes and assumptions that support sexual aggression against women and has exposed and challenged cultural myths about sexual aggression (Estep, Burt, & Milligan, 1977; Burt, 1980; Burt & Katz, 1987). Although myths still abound, feminist theory and advocacy have affected sex-offender treatment approaches significantly by enlarging the system that is viewed as dysfunctional. Sexual aggression is now viewed as a problem involving not only the personal functioning of offenders but also cultural mechanisms guiding gender identity development, gender role interaction, and standards of gender behavior.

Groth, Hobson, and Gary (1982), after treating many child sex offenders from a general psychoanalytic perspective, stated, "it would be misleading to suggest that we have reached a state of clinical knowledge that insures successful rehabilitation of adults who sexually molest children" (p. 140). They agreed that the issues involved in sexual aggression are much broader than simply individual clinical or psychological problems. Cultural, legal, political, economic, educational, medical, and spiritual concerns are involved, and effective intervention should involve all of these perspectives (Groth, 1983). Effective treatment of sexual offenders should include a variety of techniques targeted to several personal/cultural system levels, and approaches that focus exclusively on the psychodynamic functioning of the offender should not be the treatment of choice.

Behavioral Techniques

Several treatment techniques based upon classical and operant conditioning theory have been developed and used with some success. These methods of treatment are based upon the assumption that in their early development, particularly through puberty, sexual offenders learned through complicated and repetitive sequences of desensitization, reinforcement, pairing, and generalization to become sexually aroused to inappropriate stimuli such as violence, domination, pain, children, or objects (Abel et al., 1984). The goal of these intervention procedures is to eliminate these deviant sexual arousal patterns and develop or increase sexual response to appropriate and legal stimuli.

Satiation Therapy

Satiation is a procedure where a response is eliminated by repeatedly eliciting the response until the desire for the stimulus is eliminated. That is, it no longer has reinforcing properties and even takes on aversive qualities. There are two primary forms of satiation used with sex offenders, verbal and masturbatory (Marshall, 1979; Laws, 1980).

Verbal satiation may be conducted either in the laboratory with psychophysiological aids or at home. In either case, the offender is required to verbalize his deviant sexual fantasies aloud for 30 minutes or longer without stopping, while attempting to become sexual aroused. In the laboratory, he may wear a headset that is connected to a voice-operated relay such that if he pauses for more than five seconds, a loud tone goes off in his ears. The only way he can stop the irritating tone is to start speaking again. The deviant fantasy may be monitored by a therapist via intercom, or it may be tape recorded and checked later. After a period of time, the fantasy loses its sexually arousing properties. Repeated verbalization and further attempts to become aroused result in a pairing of the deviant fantasy with the inability to be sexually stimulated and extreme boredom. Laws reported, "What happens is that it blows away fantasies immediately. Within two or three weeks, or within a few sessions, the offender has totally exhausted his repertoire of effective fantasies. If he cannot think of anything to say, the tone goes off in his ears, so he has to talk, and only deviant fantasies will do" (cited in Knopp, 1984, p. 120).

A second form of satiation utilizes masturbation to achieve a similar satiated effect (Marshall, 1979; Kremsdore, Holmen, & Laws, 1979). The advantage of masturbatory satiation over verbal satiation is that the physiological responses of the orgasmic cycle are used to pair a physical inability to become aroused with the deviant sexual stimuli pattern. Using this procedure, the offender imagines and verbalizes an appropriate, nonviolent sexual scene with a consenting adult while masturbating to orgasm. Immediately after the pleasurable orgasmic response has ended, the offender switches to imagining and verbalizing a deviant sexual scene that he normally finds arousing while continuing to masturbate and attempting to become aroused. Because the offender is in the refractory period of the orgasmic cycle, it will be difficult or even impossible for him to become aroused, achieve an erection, and experience a second orgasm. The offender continues to masturbate to this deviant fantasy and seek to become aroused for 50 minutes after ejaculation. In this way, the deviant sexual fantasy is repeatedly paired with the physiological inability to become sexually aroused as well as with extreme boredom. As with covert sensitization, the verbalized fantasies are audiotaped and checked by the therapist to promote compliance and improve the offender's technique (McGuire, Carlisle, & Young, 1965). Abel and Blanchard (1974) suggested that at least 20 hours of masturbatory satiation are required to be an effective treatment.

Marshall and Barbaree (1978) reviewed other outcome research and concluded that the evidence for the effectiveness of satiation therapy was positive and suggested that it should become a standard treatment component for sex offenders. Marshall (1979) reported on two single-case design studies and stated that satiation is not only effective for reducing deviant sexual interests, but it also appears to be valuable when aversion therapy has failed. Masturbatory satiation was also a part of the successful treatment program described in Abel et al. (1984).

Covert Sensitization

Covert sensitization (CS) seeks to reduce deviant sexual arousal by repeatedly pairing sexually aberrant fantasies with highly aversive images that produce fear, anxiety, and distress. It is a procedure that "sensitizes" the offender to inappropriate stimuli and is carried out using fantasies and images rather than in vivo. Thus, it is termed "covert." Offenders begin a CS session by imagining a deviant scene that they would normally find highly sexually arousing, such as a naked child or a scene of sexual violence or rape. As they begin to become sexually aroused to the image, they immediately switch to imagining a scene they find highly aversive, such as themselves being arrested and being locked in prison or telling family members about their offense. They continue to imagine this scene until they become extremely anxious. At this point they "escape" the aversive scene by fantasizing a nondeviant, nonviolent scene of sexual activity with a consenting adult. In this way the previously sexually stimulating images acquire negative emotional properties and are no longer pleasurable. The appropriate sex scene acts as a negative reinforcer by removing the aversive scene and relieving the anxiety. Consequently, it develops positive emotional properties. A session typically consists of three cycles of fantasies, and three to four sessions per week are performed by the offender. Sessions are audiotaped by the offender and checked by the therapist to insure compliance and improve technique.

An example of the use of CS is presented in Barlow, Leitenberg, and Agras (1969). They conducted a case study in which they treated a heterosexual child molester using a form of CS. During the course of treatment, the client received descriptions of scenes in which he became nauseated when approaching a small girl but felt relieved when he turned away. An extinction phase followed in which the subject was told to stop imagining the sexually arousing scene instead of being told to imagine being nauseated. A reacquisition phase completed the study. Ratings of sexual attractiveness of deviant scenes, frequency of deviant sexual urges outside of treatment, and skin conductance responses to descriptions of selected deviant sexual scenes markedly declined during acquisition. Thus, the authors concluded that CS was a technique that deserved more extensive evaluation with clients that have the verbal skills required for imagining the aversive stimuli.

Maletzky (1980) utilized CS with 100 self-referred and court-ordered offenders. Results indicated positive results with both types of offenders at the end of treatment and up to 30 months after termination. Brownmill, Hayes, and Barlow (1977) used CS in a controlled study to eliminate child-related sexual behavior and urges, in addition to an orgasmic reconditioning procedure to increase heterosexual responsiveness. Positive changes over a six-month follow-up period were indicated by self-report and plethysmography. CS was also a primary component of the successful integrated treatment program described by Abel et al. (1984). These results suggest that CS is an effective treatment for motivated offenders who possess the cognitive and verbal skills needed to complete the procedure.

Aversion Therapy

The theoretical basis for aversion therapy is punishment and classical conditioning theory. Though the theoretical basis is the same, unlike covert sensitization, with aversion therapy an actual aversive stimulus is administered in vivo rather than covertly imagined. In aversion therapy, deviant sexual behavior (e.g., cross-dressing), visual or auditory depictions of deviant behavior or stimuli for deviant sexual arousal, or fantasies of deviant sexual stimuli and behavior are paired with and/or immediately followed by the application of a highly physically aversive stimulus. The aversive stimulus may be administered by a therapist or by the client. Chemical agents that induced nausea (McConaghy, 1969) were first used as the aversive stimulus, but they largely have been replaced by the use of foul smells (e.g., ammonia capsules) and mild electric shock (Marks & Bancroft, 1970).

An example of therapist-controlled laboratory-based aversion therapy is that a client is shown brief slide presentations of his known deviant stimuli for sexual arousal (e.g., a naked young child, a violent scene); and sexual arousal is monitored by self-report and phalleometric methods. At the peak of sexual arousal, a highly repugnant odor or a mild electric shock is administered to the client by the therapist. In this manner, the deviant stimuli lose their arousal properties; and an anxious response to them is conditioned in the client (Laws, 1981).

An example of client-controlled, home-based aversion therapy is having a client fantasize about a specific deviant sexual stimulus or situation and then sniff a small plastic film case containing a broken ammonia capsule after each short fantasy image. The cycle of fantasy-stimulus is repeated many times. As with the laboratory-based approach, the deviant stimuli quickly lose their ability to inspire sexual arousal and take on anxiety-producing qualities.

Aversion therapy has been used in the treatment of ego dystonic homosexuality (Bancroft, 1970; Feldman & MacCublloch, 1971), exhibitionism (Evans, 1970), transvestism, fetishism, pedophilia, and sadomasochism (Bancroft & Marks, 1968). Maletzky (1980) treated 38 molesters of male children by pairing aversive odors with deviant fantasies. Homework included aversive imaginal procedures, changes in masturbation fantasies, and manipulation of the environment. Based upon a nationwide search, only four legal charges in a three-year follow-up period were filed against the subjects. Quinsey, Chaplin, and Carrigan (1980) reported positive results using biofeedback and signaled punishment aversion therapy with mild electric shock as the stimulus in the treatment of 18 child molesters. Quinsey, Bergersen, and Steinman (1976) used mild electrical shock aversion therapy with 10 child molesters and reported a significant average increase in sexual preference for adults over children among the subjects. Marks, Gelder, and Bancroft (1970) utilized mild electrical shock aversion therapy with 24 sexual deviants of several types. They reported improvement with all clients except transsexuals. They concluded that despite the unpleasant nature of aversion therapy, it appears to be an effective treatment.

The use of aversion therapy, particularly therapist-controlled stimulus administration techniques, raises several ethical and professional issues for therapists treating sex offenders. The application of an actual aversive stimulus appears to violate the admonition to "first, do no harm" that all helping professions affirm. Aversion therapy also suffers from a negative public and, at times, professional perception that it is "mind control," "human experimentation" or "something out of *Clockwork Orange*." On the other hand, there are sound theoretical bases for the techniques, empirical evidence supporting their effectiveness, and no evidence that they are any more risk-prone than other commonly used treatments. Consequently, not using them means denying effective treatment to clients in need. All treatment techniques carry risks and may cause some form of temporary discomfort in order to achieve desired long-term benefits. Therefore, while the valid ethical concerns associated with aversion therapy should be carefully considered and taken into account when it is used, the techniques should not be rejected merely because they seem unpleasant. Client-controlled techniques using olfactory stimuli appear to be the most acceptable from an ethical point of view. Therapist-controlled techniques using electric shock as the stimulus, while not universally considered unacceptable, do present more ethical and professional problems and have not been found to be dramatically more effective. Consequently, when aversion therapy is indicated, client-controlled, olfactory techniques should be employed first.

Cognitive Restructuring

Abel et al. (1984) have proposed that most child molesters utilize a series of distorted cognitive beliefs in order to internally justify their sexually deviant behavior. They suggested that discrepancies between molesters' behavior and societal proscriptions against sexual aggressiveness are likely to cause them to feel a strong sense of dissonance and consequent feelings of anxiety, guilt, shame, and blame. In order to relieve this emotional distress, molesters progressively develop a set of beliefs that enable them to justify their aggressive behavior. This matrix of distorted cognitions forms an internal justification that supports their continued sexual aggression against children. Thoughts such as "The child enjoys the sexual activity," "Children can make their own decisions about having sex with an adult," "Sexual activity with an adult does not hurt the child," "Having sex with a child is a good way to teach the child about sex," and "Behavior that does not involve penetration is not really sexual" are examples of justifying cognitive distortions. This basic model of cognitive internal justification can also be applied to other types of sex offenders.

Treatment involves exposing and altering the justifying distorted cognitions and is termed cognitive restructuring. Many of the techniques used in traditional cognitive-behavioral therapy can be applied to this problem (Meichenbaum, 1977; Mahoney, 1974). Typically, treatment begins by examining beliefs that are part of other undesired but nonsexually deviant behaviors (e.g., beliefs supporting poor work habits, driving too fast, carelessness, shyness). In this manner, the process of the therapy is introduced in the context of less threatening problems. Clients are encouraged to define the undesired behavior or emotion, discuss actual incidents where they occur, examine the specific thoughts and beliefs they are thinking in those incidents that form the cognitive setting for the behavior or emotion, challenge the validity of those thoughts and beliefs, and replace them with appropriate ones. Clients are also taught to make use of feedback from the therapist and other group members in exposing and changing their beliefs.

When the clients have had successful experiences with less toxic issues, the focus is shifted to the specific problems of sexually aggressive behavior. Clients again examine specific abusive incidents and expose the thoughts and beliefs that support their behavior, including listing these thoughts in writing. The beliefs may then be challenged directly by the therapist, and more appropriate thoughts may be substituted. Abel et al. (1984) suggest using a role play procedure where the therapist plays an offender who adheres to the client's exposed beliefs and the client plays a probation officer, family member, or other figure. The offender is then put in the position of having to dispute his own beliefs. In this manner, the validity of the distorted cognition can be contested; and appropriate and valid information can be put in its place. It is common for new distorted beliefs to be exposed during the course of the restructuring therapy. The procedure is then applied to these newly discovered

is well and continues until all the major cognitive distortions
en exposed, challenged, and altered.

Training

The obvious deficits in the social behavior of many sexual offenders have prompted a number of therapists to try to teach the
offender appropriate ways of interacting with peers and appropriate
sexual partners. Explanations of why men rape or molest children
have often pointed to the poor social, assertiveness, and heterosocial skills of these individuals as a contributing factor to their aggressive behavior (Abel, Blanchard, & Becker, 1978; Quinsey,
1977). Hayes, Brownell, and Barlow (1983) defined heterosocial
skills as those behaviors necessary to interact successfully in social
and sexual interactions with a person of the opposite sex. For example, when asking for a date, a person must judge the other's interest, make "small talk," determine the appropriate time to ask, be
pleasant yet forthright, sound interested, and so forth. They suggest
that if any of these component behaviors are missing, successful
interactions are unlikely. Even if high levels of heterosexual arousal
are present, a heterosexual skills deficit could render a person in-
capable of forming a successful heterosexual relationship.

Segal and Marshall (1985) conducted a controlled study to address some of the criticisms of previous investigations of heterosexual social skills of sex offenders. First, they contended that the use
of a criterion group of low socioeconomic community-based males
while controlling for the effects of social class (Stermac & Quinsey,
1986) does not tell us whether negative results portray rapists as
equally or less skilled than the average male. Therefore, they suggest that males from high social class backgrounds be included to
correct this problem. The second criticism relates to the vast
amount of descriptive research on the issue of why men rape and
molest children that has pointed to poor heterosexual skills as possible precipitant of these behaviors (Abel, Blanchard, & Becker,
1978). More empirical research is needed to help to determine what
type of skill deficits characterize these offenders. A final criticism
offered by Segal and Marshall (1985) related to the confounding of
different types of sexual offenses, which is reflected in Barlow,

Abel, Blanchard, Bristow, and Young's (1977) research. Barlow and his colleagues compared a group of 10 sexual offenders (which comprised fetishists, exhibitionists and rapists) with 20 socially skilled males. No specificity of deficits can be inferred from their findings because the sexual offenders were composed of individuals with different sexual problems. Alexander and Johnson's (1980) research contained the same methodological flaw. A complicating factor is that many sexual offenders perform a variety of sexual offenses and paraphiliac acts (Abel et al., 1987).

In Segal and Marshall's (1985) investigation, the performance of rapists and child molesters on in vivo, questionnaire, and cognitive assessments of social skills was compared with those of inmates who were not sex offenders, as well as with nonincarcerated males of low and high socioeconomic status. Behavioral ratings provided by the subjects, confederate, and the two independent judges were consistent and portrayed low socioeconomic males as generally less skilled and more anxious than their high socioeconomic counterparts. Within the sex offender groups, child molesters presented a clearer profile of heterosexual inadequacy than did rapists. These subjects rated themselves as less skilled and more anxious in heterosexual interactions and less assertive in accepting positive feedback from others.

Sex Education

A severe lack of accurate sexual information certainly is not limited to sex offenders, and such a deficit is not viewed as a primary cause of sexually aggressive behavior. However, a lack of accurate sexual information is likely to promote avoidance of appropriate adult sexual and nonsexual relationships and general sexual insecurity. It will also act to support and provide a base of misinformation for the development of distorted cognitions about aggressive sexual behavior. Consequently, a short course that describes basic human sexual anatomy and physiology, sexual functioning, common sexual dysfunctions and disorders, sexual communication, common and appropriate sexual practices, and common sexual myths has been used as a component in many successful treatment programs. Sex education appears to be particularly useful in conjunction with different types of skill training treatment components (Abel et al., 1984; Whitman & Quinsey, 1981). Of course, sex education alone would be an entirely inadequate intervention for sexual offenders. However, it is recommended as an important component of an integrated, multicomponent treatment program.

Family-System Approaches

With the development of systems approaches to the conceptualization and treatment of emotional and behavioral problems in general, there has been a rapid increase in interest in using such an approach with sexual offenses, particularly intrafamilial child sexual abuse. A basic assumption of the family systems approach is that the sexually abusive behavior of the offender is part of a larger system of interpersonal interaction within the family, and that the interaction and relationships between family members affect and are affected by the abusive behavior. Therefore, the functioning of the whole family system and its various subsystems (marital, parent-child, and sibling) should be a primary focus of treatment. A second assumption is that the functionality of the family needs to be restored and a safe and nurturing environment needs to be established for the child.

Saunders, McClure, and Murphy (1987) assessed 49 families where the father had acknowledged sexually abusing at least one of the children. The assessment took place during the first eight weeks of a 12-month treatment program and utilized a multirespondent, multilevel empirical assessment strategy. They reported that incest families tended to be significantly more socially isolated, to be more dependent upon external organizing systems (e.g., church, work, military), to be more chaotically organized internally, to exhibit poorer executive subsystem functioning, and to have higher moral-religious emphasis than normal families. They also reported that there tends to be a strong emotional coalition between perpetrators and victims, and that nonabused siblings occupy an "outsider" role in the family. They suggested that the perpetrator-victim dyad is a controlling force in the family system to which other family members and subsystems accommodate. They concluded that the findings support the basic assumptions of the family systems treatment model suggesting that in incest families the interactions of all family members and subsystems should be taken into account in treatment.

Based upon the same study, Saunders and McClure (1987) concluded that a community-systems model of treatment involving all family members in several modalities of treatment was the treatment of choice in incest cases. They indicated that individual therapy such as behavioral interventions designed to reduce deviant sexual arousal was congruent with and should be a part of the community-systems approach.

Kroth (1979) conducted an independent analysis of the Child Abuse Treatment Program of Santa Clara County, which is based on a family-systems approach of treatment. The results indicated that there was a slightly lower but meaningful percentage of success by subjective criteria: fathers were returned to the home after a median period of 90 days, and 92% of the fathers did eventually return to their homes. Mrazek (1984) offered the caution that the outcomes in the other programs appeared to be less positive. Lanyon (1986) also states that the family-systems approach seems to be the state of the art. But he cautions that systematic research is needed to identify its effective components because it is usually very costly in terms of therapeutic time. Another empirical need is to document the extent of its success in eliminating the man's deviant sexual behaviors, thoughts and feelings.

Pharmacotherapy

The use of pharmacotherapy involving antiandrogens for sex offenders has considerable appeal for many segments of the public, but its use is controversial (e.g., Fischer, 1984). Spodak, Falck, and Rappeport (1978) concluded that clinical reports on the use of antihormone therapy have shown mixed outcomes, and side effects are reported as problematic (Langevin, 1983). The underlying philosophy of this treatment approach is that some sexual offenses are a behavioral manifestation of intense aberrant drives which represent a condition that is potentially treatable with medication. The changes (reduction in the strength of arousal) are temporary, and sexual arousal to inappropriate stimuli is reported to return when the drug is terminated (McFarland, 1986). Antihormone treatment takes immediate effect; the drug appears to be easily administered and monitored, and it is a relatively inexpensive form of treatment.

Ortmann (1980) contends that the most notable advantage of anti-hormone treatment is that it restrains sexual criminality while at the same time allowing a normal sex life. Berlin (1982) contends that the weekly injections of the drug provide the potential for compulsive offenders to curb their sexual drive and sexual fantasies through the suppression of production of the male hormone testosterone. This reduction in testosterone is perceived as increasing their capacity for self-control and diminishing "obsessive ruminations and preoccupations that they are unable to exclude from their minds." Drug therapy has been used primarily with the most compulsive paraphiliacs, namely, exhibitionists, and male pedophiles attracted to the same sex; with voyeurs, masochists, and other paraphiliacs; and least often with compulsive rapists. The injections do not create impotence but have the effect of "cooling down" the sex offender while other psychotherapeutic and behavioral interventions can be administered. In other cases, the injections may be lowered in dosage and maintained for an extended period of time.

Depo-Provera is a commonly used intramuscular injection aimed at reducing testicular testosterone production, and to returning testosterone levels of sex offenders back to pre-pubertal male levels. Behavioral and cognitive behavior therapies are almost always included as part of the treatment (McFarland, 1986). Effective rehabilitation in the treatment of sex offenders with Depo-Provera is dependent upon a careful selection of appropriate candidates. Berlin and Meinecke (1981) assert that evaluation of sex offenders must result in the diagnosis of paraphiliacs, who are characterized by recurrent, persistent fantasies about deviant sex, . . . erotic cravings perceived as noxious when frustrated, . . . and relatively stereotyped sex activity. They further stated that Depo-Provera does not treat aggression per se, but it may reduce aggression that is sex related (Berlin & Meinecke, 1981).

Researchers employing drug treatments remain enthusiastic about their potential (e.g., Berlin & Meinecke, 1981), and there is the belief that new and more sophisticated drugs such as cyproterone hold particular promise for reducing deviant but normal arousal. A middle-of-the-road position might be that at the present time, drug treatment should be considered for a small minority of offenders for whom other treatments have consistently failed or are unsuitable (Lanyon, 1986; McFarland, 1986).

Cordoba and Chapel (1983) suggest that antiandrogenic drugs offer an alternative pharmacological treatment that is biologically effective. Ortmann (1980) looked at a number of studies comparing recidivism rates of sex offenders prior to antihormone treatment and after such treatments. He found that prior to antihormone treatment, sex offenders mentioned a recidivism rate at close to 100%. In contrast, while these same sex offenders were on antihormone treatment, the recidivism rate was very low, even falling to zero.

Controversies over the use of Depo-Provera are varied. Questions have been raised about:

1. *Its short-term negative effects.* The short-range negative effects of the drug may include weight gain, sometimes up to 30 pounds. In some cases, hypertension has been reported. Other drug related complaints are hot flashes, cold sweats, and nightmares, mild elevation of blood sugar in some clients, weakness and fatigue, loss of some body hair, and tenderness in the testes because it slows or shuts off their functioning (a symptom that is reversed when Depo-Provera is discontinued (Knopp, 1984). Berlin (1982) comments that although such short-term negative side effects occur in some patients, careful monitoring is therefore required and should always be considered when deciding to use the drug.

2. *Its potential for more harmful long-range effects.* Berlin (1982) states that the long-ranged effects of Depo-Provera are difficult to pinpoint scientifically, particularly since the longest period of time humans have been receiving injections is for 10 to 15 years. According to Knopp (1984), opponents of the drug, however, fear it may be carcinogenic. Animal studies conducted by the UpJohn Company (the manufacturers) showed that doses 25 times those proposed for humans caused breast cancers in female beagle dogs. The Food and Drug Administration has approved the drug for treating inoperable cancer of the endometrium and kidney, but not specifically for the treatment of sex offenders.

3. *Its potential for use under conditions that are involuntary,*

unmonitored, and indiscriminately punitive rather than remedial. Berlin is vehemently opposed to using the drug as punishment.

4. *Its efficacy in controlling sexually aggressive behaviors.* Berlin (1982) claims an 85% success rate with the men who have gone through his program since the formulation of his program in 1979.

Surgical Procedures

Castration

The surgical removal of the testicles in sexual offenders is a procedure that is rarely used in this country on ethical grounds, but has been utilized in Europe more extensively on a voluntary basis (Lanyon, 1986). In a review of several outcome studies on the long-term effects of castration, Heim and Hursch (1979) reported that a dramatic reduction in sex offenses was a common finding. However, these studies suffered methodological flaws such as relying on self-report data and rearrest rates as outcome measures and the lack of appropriate comparison groups. Langevin (1983) indicated that sex drive was not significantly and reliably reduced by castration. He also reported a wide range of undesirable physical and psychological side effects. He concluded that sufficient empirical support is lacking for castration to be recommended as a treatment method for any type of sex offender. Heim (1981) reported on 39 voluntarily castrated sex offenders in West Germany who were released. Results indicated that frequency of coitus, masturbation, and sexual thoughts were strongly reduced after castration. However, 31% of the offenders were still able to engage in sexual intercourse. He concluded that the results do not justify castration as a reliable treatment.

The underlying premise for the use of castration as a treatment for sex offenders is that surgical removal of the sex glands will cause a diminution of sex hormones, which will result in the reduction or abolition of the sex drive and an elimination of sexual violence (Baker, 1984; Ortmann, 1980). While the evidence demonstrates that sexual drive is strongly affected by castration, it does not eliminate the ability to achieve an erection and have intercourse in a large proportion of offenders. Therefore, it appears to be an inadequate treatment. The major question that has been asked in regard to castration is whether castration of sex offenders is a treatment provided by state or merely the imposition of punitive sanctions (Baker, 1984; Heim & Hursch, 1979). Baker asserts that once treatment exceeds the cure, it is inappropriate to label such action as treatment.

Stereotaxic Hypothalamotomy

A second surgical technique that is rarely used in this country but is more common in Western and Eastern Europe is stereotaxic hypothalamotomy. In this procedure, small sections of the hypothalamus are removed or destroyed in an effort to disrupt the production of male hormonal agents, decrease the offender's ability to experience sexual arousal, and limit his impulsive tendencies. The complex interactions between the higher central nervous system functions and neuroendocrine mechanisms that are mediated by the hypothalamic-pituitary axis, the testes, and their feedback mechanisms are not well understood (Bradford, 1985). Consequently, like all psychosurgery, it is an imprecise procedure with unpredictable behavioral results.

Rieber and Sigusch (1979) reviewed the data on the stereotaxic hypothalamotomy and examined case records from 70 West German cases. They concluded that the scientific model on which the procedure is based is incomplete and that the procedures were performed on questionable scientific and clinical grounds. They stated that the procedure is highly suspect as an ethical and effective treatment for sex offenders.

DISCUSSION

While programs that treat victims of sexual assault and their families have proliferated (Giarretto, 1982; Knopp, 1984), there have been fewer advances in the treatment of sexual offenders. The reasons for the difficulty are readily recognized. Many offenders are not apprehended; they generally deny their aggressive behavior; and therapists do not like to work with this population. However, treatment of known offenders is a primary way future victimizations can be reduced.

Based upon the review presented in this article, there are some tentative conclusions that can be drawn regarding the treatment of sexual offenders. First, there now exists a variety of treatment techniques for dealing with sexual offenders, many of which have indicated some degree of success. However, more rigorous research is needed before definite claims of effectiveness can be asserted. Promising therapies include such techniques as masturbatory satiation, covert sensitization, heterosocial skills training, cognitive restructuring, and antiandrogen drug therapy.

Second, while there are controversies about the effectiveness of various approaches, the issue for many practitioners and researchers seems to be not whether any effective approaches exist, but rather how to mix and match approaches with the various types of sexual offenders in the most efficient manner (Finkelhor, 1984). A third conclusion that stems from the preceding one relates to the recognition by researchers and practitioners that treatment approaches used with sexual offenders need to be eclectic. Therefore, treatment approaches need to be amenable to individual and group counseling and need to be able to confront the total situation and personality of the sexual offender. Too often, clinicians and researchers exaggerate the importance of one or another treatment approach without having a solid practice and/or empirical foundation for their selection. For example, behavioral therapy has been promulgated as a very effective mode of treatment without the proper delineation of the diversity of its specific treatment approaches (Abel, 1978; Laws & O'Neil, 1979).

Finally, researchers and practitioners seem to agree that many sexual offenders can be treated successfully, if treatment is earlier; if assessment is complete and individualized to the offender and his offense(s); if placement is appropriate; if the treatment approaches meet the needs of the offender; if the offender accepts responsibility for the offenses and understands the sequence of thoughts, feeling, events, circumstances, and arousal stimuli that make up the "offense syndrome" that preceded his involvement in sexually assaultive behaviors; and if the offender learns how to intervene in or break into his offense pattern and call upon the appropriate methods, tools, or procedures he has learned in order to suppress, control, manage and stop the behavior (Knopp, 1984).

Given this critique of the literature on the treatment of sexual offenders, several implications are highlighted for our future efforts in this area. Studies that compare the results obtained with different treatment techniques are required to evaluate the power and effectiveness of various treatment approaches. Future research on effectiveness of treatment approaches should use experimental and control groups. Such comparative studies would be particularly informative if they were conducted with a heterogeneous, as well as homogeneous samples of sex offenders. The use of multivariate analyses in these investigations will allow us to examine the interaction between and within types of sex offenders and intervention. These interactional effects should provide a means for allowing researchers and practitioners to individualize treatment approaches and provide more rigorous empirical support on the effectiveness of singular and/or multiple treatment approaches based on the type of sexual offenses committed.

More research is also needed in the prediction of pretreatment and posttreatment assessment of sexual behavior and social functioning on the part of sex offenders. Because most of the current research on this topic has involved data that are known about the offender at the time of treatment, which is easily biased by the offender, posttreatment measures of change need to be developed as well as pretreatment measures. Additionally, multiple measures of treatment effects should be used in the evaluation of effectiveness.

Further research is needed in the area of identification of psychological, situational, behavioral, and familial correlates, as well as others that predispose the sex offender for successful or unsuccessful participation in treatment programs. This would promote successful treatment matches and allow for the development of more specialized treatment strategies which would provide a better means for evaluating and monitoring responses to treatment by sex offenders.

Sex offenders experience difficulties in many areas of their lives. Therefore, there is a need for more comprehensive treatment programs and approaches. A program of this nature should cover problems such as sexual dysfunctioning, anxiety, deficit in social and vocational skill, sex knowledge and sexual control. Consequently, researchers and policy makers should direct more attention to community treatment of sex offenders, especially in light of the fact that many offenders never serve any time for their assaultive behavior. Community programs must be developed also to attack the roots of sex assaults and to break the intergenerational cycles.

REFERENCES

Abel, G. (1978). Treatment of sexual aggressives. *Criminal Justice and Behavior, 5*, 291-293.

Abel, G., Becker, J., Cunningham-Rathner, J., Rouleau, J., Kaplan, M., & Reich, J. (1984). *The treatment of child molesters*. Atlanta, GA: Behavioral Medicine Laboratory, Emory University.

Abel, G., Becker, J., Mittleman, M., Cunningham-Rathner, J., Rouleau, J., & Murphy, W. (1987). Self-reported sex crimes of nonincarcerated paraphiliacs. *Journal of Interpersonal Violence, 2*(1), 3-25.

Abel, G., & Blanchard, E. (1974). The role of fantasy treatment of deviation. *Archives of General Psychiatry, 30*(4), 467-475.

Abel, G., Blanchard, E., & Becker, J. (1978). An integrated treatment program for rapists. In R. T. Rada (Ed.), *Clinical aspects of the rapist* (pp. 161-214). New York: Grune and Stratton.

Ageton, S. (1983). *Sexual assault among adolescents*. Lexington, MA: Lexington Books.

Albin, R. (1977). Review essay: Psychological studies of rape. *Signs: Journal of Women in Culture and Society, 3*, 423-435.

Alexander, B., & Johnson, S. (1980). Reliability of heterosocial skills measurement with sex offenders. *Journal of Behavioral Assessment, 2*, 225-237.

Alford, J., Kasper, C., & Baumann, R. (1984). Diagnostic classifications of sexual child offenders. *Corrections and Social Psychiatry, 30*(2), 40-46.

Annis, L. (1982). A residential treatment program for male sex offenders. *International Journal of Offender Therapy and Comparative Criminology, 26*(3), 223-234.

Baker, W. (1984). Castration of the male sex offender: A legally impermissible alternative. *Loyola Law Review, 30*, 377-399.

Bancroft, J. (1970). A comparative study of aversion and desensitization in the treatment of homosexuality. In L.E. Burns & J.L. Wosely (Eds.), *Behavior therapy in the 1970's*. Bristol: Wright.

Bancroft, J., & Marks, I. (1968). Electrical aversion therapy of sexual deviations. *Proceedings of the Royal Society of Medicine, 61*, 796-799.

Barlow, D., Abel, G., Blanchard, E., Bristow, A., & Young, L. (1977). A heterosocial skills behavior checklist for males. *Behavior Therapy, 8*, 229-239.

Barlow, D., Agras, W., Leitenberg, H., Callahan, E., & Moore, R. (1972). The contribution of therapeutic instruction to covert sensitization. *Behavior Research and Therapy, 10*, 411-415.

Barlow, D., Leienberg, H., & Agras, W. (1969). Experimental control of sexual deviation through manipulation of the norxious scene in covert sensitization. *Journal of Abnormal Psychology, 74*, 596-601.

Becker, J., Cunningham-Rathner, J., & Kaplan, M. (1986). Adolescent sexual offenders: Demographics, criminal and sexual histories, and recommendations for reducing future offenses. *Journal of Interpersonal Violence, 1*(4), 431-445.

Berlin, F. (1982). Sex offenders: A biomedical perspective. In J. Grier & I. Stuart (Eds.), *Sexual aggression: Current perspectives on treatment* (Vol *1*). New York: Van Nostrand Reinhold.

Berlin, F., & Meinecke, C. (1981). Treatment of sex offenders with antiandrogenic medication: Conceptualization, review of treatment modalities, and preliminary findings. *American Journal of Psychiatry, 138*(5), 601-607.

Bradford, J. (1985). Organic treatments for the male sexual offender. *Behavioral Sciences & the Law, 3*(4), 355-375.

Brownell, K., Hayes, S., & Barlow, D. (1977). Patterns of appropriate and deviant sexual arousal: The behavioral treatment of multiple sexual deviations. *Journal of Consulting and Clinical Psychology, 45*, 1144-1155.

Brownmiller, S. (1975). *Against our will: Men, women, and rape*. New York: Simon and Schuster.

Burgess, A., & Holmstrom, L. (1974). *Rape: Victims of crisis*. Bowie, MD: Robert J. Bradly.

Burt, M. (1980). Cultural myths and supports for rape. *Journal of Personality and Social Psychology, 38*(2), 217-230.

Burt, M., & Katz, B. (1987). Dimensions of recovery from rape: Focus on growth and outcomes. *Journal of Interpersonal Violence, 2*(1), 57-81.

Callahan, E., & Leitenberg, H. (1973). Aversion therapy for sexual deviation: Contingent shock and covert sensitization. *Journal of Abnormal Psychology, 81*, 60-73.

Caprio, F. (1972). Hypnosis in the treatment of sexual problems. *Hypnosis Quarterly, 17*, 10-14.

Clark, L., & Lewis, D. (1977). *Rape: The price of coercive sexuality*. Toronto, Ontario, Canada: The Women's Press.

Clark, M. (1986, May). Missouri's sexual offender program. *Corrections Today, 48*(3), 84,85,89.

Cohn, R. (1966). The sexual fantasies of the psychotherapist and their use in psychotherapy. *Journal of Sex Research, 2*, 219-226.

Cordoba, O., & Chapel, J. (1983). Medroxyprogesterone acetate antiandrogen treatment of hypersexuality in pedophiliac sex offender. *American Journal of Psychiatry, 140*(8), 1036-1039.

Crown, S. (1983). Psychotherapy of sexual deviation. *British Journal of Psychiatry, 143*, 242-247.

Dreiblatt, I. (1982, May). *Issues in the evaluation of the sex offender*. Paper presented to the Washington State Psychological Association meeting.

Estep, R., Burt, M., & Milligan, H. (1977). The socialization of sexual identity. *Journal of Marriage and the Family, 39*(1), 99-112.

Evans, D. (1970). Subjective variables and treatment effects in aversion therapy. *Behavior Research and Therapy, 8,* 147-152.

Federal Bureau of Investigation. (1986). *Crime in the United States: Uniform crime reports.* Washington, DC: U.S. Department of Justice.

Feldman, M., & MacCulloch, M. (1971). *Homosexual behavior: Therapy and assessment.* Oxford: Pergamon Press.

Ferenczi, S. (1926). *Further contribution to the theory and techniques of psychoanalysis.* J. I. Sutie, L. Woolf, & V. Woolf, (trans.). London: The Institute of Psychoanalysis. (Original work published 1924)

Finkelhor, D. (1984). *Child sexual abuse: New theory and research. Implications for Theory, Research and Practice* (pp. 221-236). New York: The Free Press.

Fischer, K. (1984, May). Old attitudes slow treatment gains for sex offenders. *APA Monitor,* 23-24.

Foote, W., & Laws, D. (1981). A daily alternative procedure for orgasmic reconditioning with a pedophile. *Journal of Behavior Therapy and Experimental Psychiatry, 12,* 267-273.

Freeman-Longo, R. (1986). The impact of sexual victimization of males. Sixth International Congress of the International Society for Prevention of Child Abuse and Neglect. *Child Abuse and Neglect, 10*(3), 411-414.

Freeman-Longo, R., & Walls, R. (1986, March). Changing a lifetime of sexual crime. *Psychology Today, 20*(3), 58-64.

Gebhard, D., Gagnon, J., Pomery, W., & Christenson, C. (1965). *Sex offenders: An analysis of types.* New York: Harper and Row.

Groth, A. (1979). *Men who rape: The psychology of the offender.* New York: Plenum Press.

Groth, A. (1983). *Juvenile and adult sex offenders: Creating a community response.* A training lecture sponsored by the Tompkins County Sexual Abuse Task Force, Ithaca, New York, June 16-17.

Groth, A., Hobson, W., & Gary, T. (1982). The child molester: Clinical observation. In J. Conte & D. Shore (Eds.), *Social work and child sexual abuse.* New York: Haworth.

Grunfeld, B., & Noreik, K. (1986). Recidivism among sex offenders: A follow-up study of 541 Norwegian sex offenders. *International Journal of Law and Psychiatry, 9,* 95-102.

Hartman, V. (1965). Group psychotherapy with sexually deviant offenders (pedophiles)—the peer group as an instrument of mutual control. *Criminal Law Quarterly, 7,* 464-479.

Hawton, K. (1983). Behavioral approaches to the management of sexual deviations. *The British Journal of Psychiatry, 143,* 248-255.

Hayes, S., Brownell, K., & Barlow, D. (1983). Heterosocial skills training and covert sensitization. Effects on social skills and sexual arousal in sexual deviants. *Behavior Research and Therapy, 21*(4), 383-392.

Heim, N. (1981). Sexual behavior of castrated sex offenders. *Archives of Sexual Behavior, 10*(1), 11-19.

Heim, N., & Hursch, C. (1979, May). Castration for sex offenders: Treatment or punishment? A review and critique of recent European literature. *Archives of Sexual Behavior*, 281.

Hobbs, M. (1980). Group therapy with sexual offenders. *Australian Journal of Clinical Hypnotherapy, 1*(2), 105-111.

Johnson, A. (1980). On the prevalence of rape in the United States. *Signs: Journal of Women in Culture and Society, 6*, 136-146.

Josiassen, R., Fantuzzo, J., & Rosen, A. (1980). Treatment of pedophilia using multistage Aversion therapy and social skills training. *Journal of Behavior Therapy and Experimental Psychiatry, 11*, 55-61.

Karpman, B. (1954). *The sexual offender and his offenses.* New York: Julian Press.

Kelley, R. (1982). Behavioral reorientation of pedophilies: Can it be done? *Clinical Psychological Review, 2*, 387-408.

Kilmann, R., Sabalis, R., Gearing, M., Bukstel, L., & Scovern, A. (1982). The treatment of sexual paraphilias: A review of the outcome research. *Journal of Sex Research, 18*, 193-252.

Kilpatrick, D., Best, C., Veronen, L., Amick, A., Villeponteaux, L., & Ruff, G. (1985). Mental health correlates of criminal victimization: A random community survey. *Journal of Consulting and Clinical Psychology, 53*, 866-873.

Kilpatrick, D., Veronen, L., Saunders, B., Best, C., Amick-McMullan, A., & Paduhovich, J. (1987). *The psychological impact of crime: A study of randomly surveyed crime victims.* Final report, NIJ Grant No. 84-IJ-CX-0039. Washington, DC: National Institute of Justice.

Kilpatrick, D., Saunders, B., Veronen, L., Best, C., & Von, J. (1987). Criminal victimization: Lifetime prevalence, reporting to police, and psychological impact. *Crime & Delinquency, 33*(4), 479-489.

Knopp, F. (1976). *Instead of prisons.* Syracuse, NY: Safer Society Press.

Knopp, F. (1984). *Retraining adult sex offenders: Methods and models.* Syracuse, NY: Safer Society Press.

Kopp, S. (1962). The character structure of sex offenders. *American Journal of Psychotherapy, 16*, 64-70.

Koss, M. (1985). The hidden rape victim: Personality, attitudinal, and situational characteristics. *Psychology of Women Quarterly, 9*, 193-212.

Koss, M., Gidycz, C., & Wisniewski, N. (1987). The scope of rape: Incidence and prevalence of sexual aggression and victimization in a national sample of higher education students. *Journal of Consulting and Clinical Psychology, 55*(2), 162-170.

Koss, M., Leonard, K., Beezley, D., & Oros, C. (1985). Nonstranger sexual aggression: A discriminant analysis of the psychological characteristics of undetected offenders. *Sex Roles, 12*, 981-992.

Koss, M., & Oros, C. (1982). Sexual Experiences Survey: A research instrument investigating sexual aggression and victimization. *Journal of Consulting and Clinical Psychology, 50*, 455-457.

Kremsdore, R., Holmen, M., & Laws, D. (1979). Case histories and shorter communications. *Behavioral Research and Therapy, 18*, 203-207.

Kroth, J. (1979). Family therapy impact on intra-familial child sexual abuse. *Child Abuse and Neglect, 3,* 297-302.

Langevin, R. (1983). *Sexual strands.* Hillsdale, NJ: Erlbaum.

Lanyon, R. (1986). Theory and treatment in child molestation. *Journal of Consulting and Clinical Psychology, 54*(2), 176-182.

Laws, D. (1980). Treatment of bisexual pedophilia by a biofeedback-assisted self-control procedure. *Behavior Research and Therapy, 18,* 207-211.

Laws, D., & O'Neil, J. (1979). *Variation on masturbatory conditioning.* Paper presented at the Second National Conference on Evaluation and Treatment of Sexual Aggressives. New York, 1979.

Lorand, A., & Balint, M. (Eds.). (1956). *Perversions: Psychodynamics and therapy.* New York: Random House.

Mahoney, M. (1974). *Cognition and behavior modification.* Cambridge, MA: Ballinger Publishing Co.

Maletsky, B. (1980). Self-referred versus court-referred sexually deviant patients: Success with assisted covert sensitization. *Behavior Therapy, 11*(3), 306-314.

Margolin, L. (1983). A treatment model for the adolescent sex offender. *Journal of Offender Counseling Services & Rehabilitation, 8*(1-2), 1-12.

Marks, I., & Bancroft, J. (1970). Sexual deviants two years after electrical aversion. *British Journal of Psychiatry, 117,* 173-185.

Marks, I., Gelder, M., & Bancroft, J. (1970). Sexual deviants two years after electric aversion. *British Journal of Psychiatry, 117,* 173-185.

Marshall, W. (1979). Satiation therapy: A procedure for reducing deviant sexual arousal. *Journal of Applied Behavior Analysis, 12,* 377-389.

Marshall, W., & Barbaree, H. (1978). The reduction of deviant arousal: Satiation treatment for sexual aggressors. *Criminal Justice and Behavior, 5*(4), 294-303.

Marshall, W., & McKnight, R. (1975). An integrated treatment program for sexual offenders. *Canadian Psychiatric Association Journal, 20,* 133-138.

Matek, O. (1985-1986). The use of fantasy training as a therapeutic process in working with sexual offenders. *Journal of Social Work & Human Sexuality, 4*(1/2), 109-123.

McCahill, T., Meyer, L., & Fischman, A. (1979). *The aftermath of rape.* Lexington, MA: Lexington Books.

McConaghy, N. (1969). Subjective and penile plethysmograph responses following aversion -- relief and apomorphine aversion therapy for homosexual impulses. *British Journal of Psychiatry, 115,* 723-730.

McFarland, L. (1986). Depo-provera therapy as an alternative to imprisonment. *Houston Law Review, 30,* 377-399.

McGuire, R., Carlisle, J., & Young, B. (1965). Sexual deviants as conditioned behavior. *Behavior Research and Therapy, 2,* 185-190.

Meichenbaum, D. (1977). *Cognitive-behavior modification: An integrative approach.* New York: Plenum Press.

Mrazek, F. (1984). Sexual abuse of children. In B. Lahey and A. Karzdin (Eds.),

Advances in child clinical psychology (Vol. 6, pp. 199-215). New York: Plenum Press.

Ortmann, B. (1980). The treatment of sexual offenders. *International Journal of Legal Psychiatry, 3,* 443-450.

Peters, J., Pedigo, J., Steg, J., & McKenna, J. (1968). Group psychotherapy of the sex offender. *Federal Probation, 32,* 41-45.

Peters, S., Wyatt, G., & Finkelhor, D. (1986). Prevalence. In D. Finkelhor (Ed.), *A sourcebook on child sexual abuse.* Beverly Hills, CA: Sage Publications.

Quinsey, V. (1977). The assessment and treatment of child molesters: A review. *Canadian Psychological Review, 18*(3), 204-220.

Quinsey, V., Bergersen, S., & Steinman, C. (1976). Changes in physiological and verbal responses of child molesters during aversion therapy. *Canadian Journal of Behavioural Science, 8*(2), 202-212.

Quinsey, V., Chaplin, T., & Carrigan, W. (1980). Biofeedback and signaled punishment in the modification of inappropriate sexual age preferences. *Behavior Therapy, 11*(4), 567-576.

Rapaport, K., & Burkhart, B. (1984). Personality and attitudinal characteristics of sexually coercive college males. *Journal of Abnormal Psychology, 93,* 216-221.

Resnick, H., & Peters, J. (1967). Outpatient group therapy with convicted pedophiles. *International Journal of Group Psychotherapy, 7,* 211-213.

Rieber, I., & Sigusch, V. (1979). Psychosurgery on sex offenders and sexual "deviants" in West Germany. *Archives of Sexual Behavior, 8*(6), 523-527.

Riemann, F. (1968). Psychoanalysis for perversions. *Zeitschrift fur Psychosomatische Medizin und Psychoanalyse, 14*(1), 3-15.

Roether, H., & Peters, J. (1972). Cohesiveness and hostility in group therapy. *American Journal of Psychiatry, 128*(8), 1014-1017.

Romero, J., & Williams, L. (1983). Group psychotherapy and intensive probation supervision with sex offenders: A comparative study. *Federal Probation, 47*(4), 36-42.

Russell, D. (1975). *The politics of rape: The victim's perspective.* New York: Stein & Day.

Russell, D. (1984). *Sexual exploitation: Rape, child sexual abuse, and workplace harassment.* Beverly Hills, CA: Sage Publications.

Sacerdote, P. (1967). *Induced dreams.* New York: Gaus.

Saunders, B., & McClure, S. (1987, September). *Marital and family system functioning among incest families: Clinical and case management implications.* Paper presented at Social Work '87, the annual meeting of the National Association of Social Workers, New Orleans, LA.

Saunders, B., McClure, S., & Murphy, S. (1987, July). *Structure, function, and symptoms in father-child sexual abuse families: A multilevel-multirespondent empirical assessment.* Paper presented at the National Family Violence Research Conference, Durham, NH.

Saunders, B., McClure, S., & Murphy, S. (1986). *Final report: Profile of incest perpetrators indicating treatability—Part I.* Washington, DC: U.S. Department of the Navy, Family Support Program.

Saunders, B., Villeponteaux, L., Kilpatrick, D., & Veronen, L. (1987, September). *Child sexual assault as a risk factor in mental health.* Paper presented at Social Work '87, the annual meeting of the National Association of Social Workers, New Orleans, LA.

Segal, Z., & Marshall, W. (1985). Heterosexual social skills in a population of rapists and child molesters. *Journal of Consulting and Clinical Psychology, 53*(1), 55-63.

Silberman, E. (1980). *Criminal violence, criminal justice.* New York: First Vintage Books.

Spanos, N. (1971). Goal directed fantasy and the performance of hypnotic test suggestion. *Psychiatry, 34,* 86-96.

Spodak, M., Falck, Z., & Rappeport, J. (1978). The hormonal treatment of paraphilias with depo-provera. *Criminal Justice and Behavior, 5,* 304-311.

Stava, L. (1984). The use of hypnotic uncovering techniques in the treatment of pedophilia: A brief communication. *The International Journal of Clinical and Experimental Hypnosis, 32*(4), 350-355.

Stermac, L., & Quinsey, V. (1986). Social competence among rapists. *Journal of Behavioral Assessment, 8*(2), 171-185.

Veronen, L., & Kilpatrick, D. (1980). Self-reported fears of rape victims: A preliminary investigation. *Behavior Modification, 4*(3), 383-396.

Watkins, J. (1971). The affect bridge: A hypnoanalytic technique. *International Journal of Clinical and Experimental Hypnosis, 19,* 21.

West, D., Roy, C., & Nichols, F. (1978). *Understanding sexual attacks.* London: Heinemann Educational Books.

Whitman, W., & Quinsey, V. (1981). Heterosocial skill training for institutionalized rapists and child molesters. *Canadian Journal of Behavioural Sciences, 13,* 105-114.

Wong, S., Gaydos, G., & Fuqua, R. (1982). Operant control of pedophilia: Reducing approaches to children. *Behavior Modification, 6,* 73-84.

Mentally Retarded Sex Offenders: Fact, Fiction, and Treatment

Robert F. Schilling
Steven P. Schinke

SUMMARY. Normal sexual functioning has only recently become a prerogative of mentally retarded persons. More often, the sexuality of women and men with mental handicaps has been viewed as deviant and as cause for concern, restrictive policies, and clinical intervention. This paper critically evaluates scientific evidence for and against mentally retarded persons' increased risk of committing sexual offenses. Etiological theories of sexual offenses among the target population are discussed in detail. In addition, the authors describe treatment strategies for mentally retarded sexual offenders. Finally, the paper gives directions for future behavioral and social science research on issues concerning sexual offenses among mentally retarded persons.

Only in recent years have professionals, advocacy groups, and parents recognized the normalcy of sexual functioning among mentally retarded persons (Craft & Craft, 1981; Edmonson, McCombs, & Wish, 1979). Even so, the sexual liberation of mentally disabled women and men is not widely approved (Heshusius, 1982; Johnson, 1984; Zetlin & Turner, 1985). Mentally retarded persons continue to be excessively vulnerable to sexual exploitation (Haywood, 1981; Schilling & Schinke, 1984). Surprisingly, the likelihood that mentally retarded persons will commit sexual offenses has received relatively little attention. This paper considers the possibility that, under some circumstances, mentally retarded persons may commit acts of sexual misconduct.

The authors thank Carla Hansen, Jeff Snow, and Charlotte Smallwood. Funding was by Grant 90CA902 from the National Center on Child Abuse and Neglect, Administration for Children, Youth, and Families, Office of Human Development Services, Department of Health and Human Services.

33

The authors begin with a discussion of prejudice and controversy about the sexual rights of mentally retarded persons. Consequently, the extent to which preconceived notions may cloud reasoned consideration of a link between mental retardation and sexual abuse is reviewed. Etiological theories of sexual assault are noted, as are implications for mentally retarded adolescents and adults. Next, evidence of sexual abuse by mentally handicapped persons is reviewed, followed by arguments that support or discredit the notion that mentally retarded persons may sexually abuse others. The authors describe efforts to treat mentally retarded offenders and outline areas for research.

SEXUALITY AND MENTAL RETARDATION

The United States allows considerably more freedom of sexual expression than many cultures permit. But this society has been less tolerant of sexual behavior on the part of mentally retarded persons. Until recently, parents and other caregivers preferred not to consider the sexual needs of mentally retarded persons. Fortunately, advocates, parents, educators, and social workers increasingly recognize that if persons with mental handicaps are to lead fuller, less protected lives, they will also have more complete sex lives than in the past.

Controversy

Societal changes notwithstanding, issues concerning sexuality and mentally retarded persons are still controversial (Brantlinger, 1983; Johnson, 1984). Few people do not have an opinion about the sexuality of persons with mental handicaps (Brantlinger, 1983). The boundaries of opinion are framed by the following positions.

Strong Advocacy. Advocates have stated that mentally retarded persons have a right to sexuality. According to some advocates, mentally retarded persons have been denied their right to be sexual because nonhandicapped persons find sex between such persons to be offensive. Defenders of this position believe that this right extends to explicit instruction in sexual techniques. Implicit in the strong-advocacy position is the belief that sexuality is a necessary part of being human.

Moderated Advocacy. Many parents and professionals believe that mentally handicapped persons should be exposed to knowledge about sexuality, and that dating, sometimes under supervision, should not be discouraged. Inappropriate public sexual expression, unplanned pregnancy, and exploitation are seen as potential problems. Parents and caregivers may deal with such concerns either by discouraging high-risk activities or by preparing developmentally disabled dependents for situations requiring sexual competence. Sexual intercourse is not necessarily encouraged, but family members and residential supervisors accept that sexual intimacy may occur.

Value-Free Position. Proponents of this view believe that sexuality is a private matter, and that policy makers and practitioners have no legitimate interest in the sexuality of mentally retarded persons. Moreover, sexual activity may not be desired by or appropriate for all persons. Sex education courses should be available, but mentally handicapped persons should be neither encouraged to engage in any kind of sexual practice nor discouraged from doing so. Although seemingly difficult to fault, the value-free position ignores the reality that sexuality presents special challenges and risks for mentally retarded persons.

Negative Position. An unknown but large proportion of Americans still believe that mentally retarded persons should not engage in sexual conduct. Because this position has few outspoken professional adherents, its logical underpinnings are not articulated in the literature. Apparently, some persons believe that sexuality is but one of many freedoms that should not be extended to developmentally disabled persons. Others believe that mentally retarded persons have excessive sex drives that must be curbed (Gross, 1985; Heshusius, 1982). Still others find public displays of affection between retarded persons offensive. Finally, concerns about the child-rearing abilities of mentally retarded parents and fears about the genetic potential of their children are associated with strong negative beliefs about the sexuality of mentally retarded persons.

Implications for Sexual Offenders

The positions outlined above offer evidence that society is struggling with issues involving mentally retarded persons and "normal'' sexuality. Sexual deviance among mentally retarded persons remains poorly understood. Before discussing the nature and extent of sexual offenses among mentally retarded persons, the authors advance three suppositions. The first of these is that social circumstances, not biological considerations, account for any differences in the sexual offense rates of retarded and nonretarded persons. Second, there is little reason to assume that mentally retarded persons in general are more likely to commit sexual abuse than nonhandicapped persons. Third, the issue of sexual abuse by persons with mental handicaps must be approached with care, as such persons are themselves vulnerable.

NATURE AND SCOPE

Sexual Offenses Defined

Sexual deviance includes a range of behavior. Some deviant behavior may not involve a violation of public standards or abuse an individual's rights. For example, certain fetishes or transvestite practices are not generally of concern to society because they occur behind closed doors or are not viewed as a threat to another individual.

In contrast, other sexual phenomena, such as rape, are clearly offenses against individuals. Still other sexual conduct, such as public disrobing, violates community standards of decency rather than the rights of a single victim. Although comprehensive typologies are available (Abel, Rouleau, & Cunningham-Rathner, 1985), an uncomplicated classification scheme will suffice for the purposes of the present discussion. Any simple classification of sexual offenses is necessarily imprecise and reflects legal rather than diagnostic nomenclature (Knopp, 1984).

Rape. Narrowly defined, this term refers to the act of forcing another person to submit to vaginal or anal intercourse, or other sex act. As used here, rape requires the use or threat of violence.

Molestation. In most instances, molestation involves children or other dependents who are unable to protect themselves from the sexual advances of an older or stronger person. An imprecise term, molestation may include fondling, rape, or frottage. A similar, though equally vague, term is "indecent liberties."

Exposure. Exhibitionists derive pleasure from exposing their genitals to others. Other "hands-off" offenses include peeping, stealing underwear, and making obscene phone calls.

Incest. This term refers to sexual contact between members of the same family. In most instances, incest involves a child and a parent, older sibling, or other relative. Sexual offenders often have a history of being incest victims and, in turn, may be involved in sexual exploitation both within and outside of the home. Incest was once considered entirely different from other sexual offenses. It has recently been suggested, however, that some forms of incest may be convenient offenses committed by victimizers who take advantage of the safety of the home and the power of their familial relationship (Becker, Kaplan, Cunningham-Rathner, & Kavoussi, 1986).

Clearly different from the victim's standpoint, these sexual offenses may or may not have distinct etiologies. Moreover, each category subsumes a number of different forms and degrees of sexual deviance. Official statistics typically categorize offenders according to these or similar gross categories that provide no information about the situational context of the sexual conduct.

Causation

Lanyon (1986) contrasted traditional and newer conceptualizations of sexual deviation. The classic view is that all sexual deviations are etiologically and theoretically similar, representing a form of character disorder. A more recent, but by no means universally accepted, view is essentially atheoretical. Proponents of this school of thought make no assumptions about causation and tend to rely on empirically derived, behavioral interventions. Neither point of view is necessarily inconsistent with the notion that developmental disabilities and sexual deviance may be linked. However, theories that rely on underlying causality are difficult to apply, because mentally retarded persons are often unable to complete psychological tests or provide reliable interview data. Although comprehensive theories have not yet evolved, evidence that sheds light on the issue of sexual deviance among mentally retarded persons should be considered from a theoretical perspective.

DIRECT EVIDENCE

Recent evidence of the extent to which mentally retarded persons may commit sexual offenses comes from a study of mentally retarded offenders. A survey of adults in Washington State correctional facilities turned up 155 subjects who met federally established criteria for developmental disability (Gross, 1985). Of these identified cases, nearly half (72) were incarcerated for sexual assault. Of 78 prisoners with IQs below 70, 33 had been convicted of sexual offenses. The same report also examined felony arrest records of 63 mentally retarded persons on developmental disabilities case loads. As with mentally retarded felons in Washington State prisons, the most frequent crimes were sexual offenses. Some 35% of those with felony arrests had been apprehended for sexual assault. Finally, the survey identified 154 persons with felony records in state institutions for developmentally disabled persons. In this group of offenders, 21% had been convicted of sexual crimes. These results strongly indicate that if a mentally retarded person is arrested for a felony, the offense is frequently sexual in nature.

Other data, also from the state of Washington, lend modest support to the findings of the above study. Landesman-Dwyer and Sulzbacher (1981) studied 210 developmentally disabled clients who were returned to institutions after failing to adjust to community living. Reasons given to explain the need for reinstitutionalization included inappropriate nudity (6), constant masturbation (4), and sexual aggression (17). Although the total of 27 sexually related reasons is not insignificant, physical aggression toward people and property, medical problems, and client incompatibility accounted for 142 of 220 responses, a much larger proportion. It should also be noted that nudity and masturbation are not offenses if they occur within a private residence.

A review of studies of mentally retarded sex offenders (Murphy, Coleman, & Abel, 1983) found that most research does not point toward higher rates of sexual offenses among mentally retarded populations. Even exhibitionists, who fit the common stereotype of the mentally retarded sexual offender, were not found to have low IQs. Together, these data provide no clear answer as to whether mentally retarded persons are more likely than nonretarded persons to commit sexual offenses.

INDIRECT EVIDENCE

Although empirical research directly focusing on the sexual offenses of mentally retarded persons is scarce, other data are informative. The social circumstances and behavioral correlates of mental retardation may provide clues about the situational specificity of undesirable sexual activity of some mentally retarded persons.

Arguments Favoring Increased Risk

Mentally Retarded Persons and Sex Offenders. Although the biases of the legal system against poor and unsophisticated offenders cannot be overlooked, criminal behavior is associated with low intelligence (Haskins & Friel, 1972; Santamour & West, 1979). Because less intelligent offenders are likely to be less skillful at avoiding detection than others, they will be apprehended more frequently than nonhandicapped persons, even though they may have the same rates of misconduct. Still, a compatible hypothesis is that mentally retarded offenders fail to consider the consequences of their actions. Persons who are mentally retarded have many of the same limitations in life skills as sex offenders. Sexual offenders and mentally retarded persons are sexually naive, socially isolated, and prefer the company of younger children (Fehrenbach, Smith, Monastersky, & Deisher, 1986; Schilling, Schinke, Blythe, & Barth, 1982; Shoor, Speed, & Bartelt, 1966). Contrary to the notion that sexual crime is etiologically distinct from other forms of social deviance, sexual offenders typically have histories of delinquent behavior (Fehrenbach, Smith, Monastersky, & Deisher, 1986; Jackson, 1984). Sex offenders and mentally retarded persons often have been sexually abused themselves, in both institutional and familial settings (Fehrenbach, Smith, Monastersky, & Deisher, 1986; Johnson, 1984; Schilling & Schinke, 1984). Because of their own experience as victims and their proximity to other vulnerable persons, mentally retarded persons in group living arrangements may inflict sexual harm on others.

Other Factors. Other possible contributing causes of sexual delinquency among mentally retarded persons are lack of knowledge about sex, limited experience in socially desirable sexual conduct, and a lack of opportunities to engage in appropriate sexual contact. Masturbation, a normal sexual outlet for most people, may be discouraged by parents and other caregivers. Dating between mentally retarded persons may be restricted or closely supervised. Thus, it is possible that the societal proscription intended to prevent undesirable sexual conduct among mentally retarded persons actually encourages the commission of sexual offenses.

Arguments Against Increased Risk

Characteristics that limit mentally retarded persons' participation in society may also limit their opportunity to commit sexual offenses. Biology, roles, and mobility merit consideration as intervening factors.

Biological Considerations. Although some aggressive sexual behavior may have biological foundation, the role of biology as an etiological contributor to sexuality remains poorly understood (Berlin, 1983; Knopp, 1984). Sexual development is often delayed in mentally retarded persons, and libido is thought to be diminished among persons with severe or profound mental retardation (Murphy, Coleman, & Abel, 1983; Robinson & Robinson, 1976). Albeit weighted with institutionalized samples, most studies of mentally retarded adults find low or unremarkable rates of reproduction (Floor, Baxter, Rosen, & Zisfein, 1975; Reed & Anderson, 1973; Schilling, Schinke, Blythe, & Barth, 1982). A reasonable but untested assumption is that sexual functioning is reduced along with most other functions in severely and profoundly retarded populations. In sum, there is little biological evidence to support the notion that mentally retarded persons are "oversexed," and at least some evidence that a portion of the mentally retarded population has lowered sex drive.

Roles. Mentally retarded persons tend to have restricted roles that may reduce their opportunity to commit certain kinds of sexual offenses. For example, mentally retarded persons are less apt than nonretarded persons to be parents or employers, or to hold other positions of trust and power. They are likely to have few dating opportunities. Thus it is plausible that mentally retarded persons would be less likely than the general population to be perpetrators of incest, sexual harassment on the job, and date rape.

Mobility. Persons who are mentally retarded are apt to be closely supervised, without their own transportation, and scrutinized by mistrustful strangers. These conditions make for reduced opportunities to commit sexual offenses. Though difficult to support empirically, it is reasonable to assume that persons with reduced roles and freedoms will have reduced opportunities to become involved in at least some kinds of sexual offenses.

These data and observations concerning the sexuality of mentally retarded persons are subject to multiple interpretations. No undeniable evidence points toward increased or decreased risk of sexual offenses by mentally retarded persons. The most convincing data, based on prison and institutional records, suggest that if mentally retarded persons are apprehended for crimes, those crimes are likely to be sexual offenses. Thus it is fair to state that sexual offenses are a legitimate concern for policy makers and practitioners who serve mentally retarded persons. Although the overall sexual offense rates of mentally retarded populations have not been established, it is likely that certain characteristics of mental retardation may translate into increased risk of some kinds of sexual offenses. Even if mentally retarded persons as a group pose no inordinate risk to potential victims of sexual assault, the few that do commit sexual offenses may require special treatment.

TREATMENT

Leaving aside the superiority of preventive approaches, treatments are needed to prepare mentally retarded offenders for lives free of sexual misconduct. The best approaches should combine interventions designed for sex offenders in general with strategies that address the particular requirements and limitations of developmentally disabled populations. Ideal treatment programs would redesign interventions so that mentally retarded persons understand the content of material that focuses on sexual behavior. In addition, postrelease monitoring, life skills training, and community supports must be tailored to fit the unique risks and needs of mentally retarded persons.

At least 643 individuals and agencies treat sex offenders; of these, 148 and 136 respectively provide services for mentally retarded adults and adolescents (Knopp, Rosenberg, & Stevenson, 1986). That such programs are concentrated in only a few states is evidence of their innovativeness. One such model is operated by the Social Skills Unit of the Correctional Treatment Program at Oregon State Hospital (Knopp, 1984). This program provides treatment for low-functioning sex offenders with less than a fourth-grade education. The goals and overarching methods of the special unit are the same as those developed for nonhandicapped offenders. Specifically, residents examine and accept responsibility for their own behavior, learn how to change their conduct, develop skills for living, and continue to receive consistent treatment in the community. Merging elements of cognitive restructuring used with offenders in general (Yochelson & Samenow, 1977) and Rational Emotive Therapy (Ellis, 1970), the originators of the program have pioneered methods that show promise for use with mentally retarded sex offenders. Relying less on insight than do other programs, the Social Skills Unit teaches offenders to label danger signals that trigger escape mechanisms. For example, one participant with a long history of molestation learned to label children "those brats," and this phrase cued him to leave the area.

Although the program remains unevaluated, the originators believe that low-functioning offenders may have a better prognosis than other sex offenders. Mentally retarded offenders may not have the sophisticated and ingrained fantasies and the associate excitement of planning the act. This intriguing hypothesis awaits investigation.

Murphy, Coleman, and Haynes (1983) have provided one of the few published discussions of interventions with mentally retarded sex offenders. Although formal protocols have not been established, the authors describe a number of issues and treatments that apply to offenders with limited cognitive abilities. They emphasize that mentally retarded persons may have a range of problems, such as aggressivity and temper tantrums, that may require behavioral or environmental intervention. Social-skill limitations and the inability to discriminate between deviant and appropriate behavior are other areas that challenge treatment providers. Mentally retarded offenders are amenable to the same kinds of treatments used with nonretarded sex offenders, including electrical aversion, satiation, and covert sensitization. However, procedures must begin at low levels, provide concrete explanations, repeat instructions frequently, and use simple language. For example, during penile assessment to determine the subject's arousal to sexual stimuli, retarded offenders are asked "Is it hard?" rather than "What percent erect are you?" As with almost all clinical work with mentally retarded offenders, the efficacy of these strategies has yet to be determined.

NEEDED RESEARCH

Description

This discussion and review of mentally retarded sexual offenders demonstrates that research in this area is sorely lacking. Although the sexuality of mentally retarded persons has received considerable attention in recent years (e.g., de la Cruz & La Veck, 1973; Gochros & Gochros, 1977; Timmers, DuCharme, & Jacob, 1981), little is known about the extent to which intellectual deficits may predispose mentally retarded persons toward sexual deviance. Studies should focus on the nature and circumstances of sexual offenses committed by mentally retarded persons. For instance, it was observed earlier that date rape is unlikely to be committed by mentally retarded persons who have restricted opportunities to date. Other kinds of sexual offenses may be more prevalent among mentally retarded persons living in group settings.

Because studies of apprehended offenders are likely to include a disproportionate number of individuals who are unskilled in avoiding detection, arrest, and prosecution, conclusions based on institutionalized or arrested populations will always be subject to criticism. Investigators should therefore also attend to the full range of sexual behavior exhibited by mentally retarded persons. Parents, residential supervisors, caseworkers, and clinicians are a rich and largely untapped source of such knowledge. By collecting data on sexual behavior — both deviant and normative — researchers will begin to understand sexual offenses within the context of sexual behavior of mentally retarded persons in general (Edgerton & Dingman, 1964). For example, precursors of illegal sexual conduct may or may not be the same for retarded and nonretarded populations. Certain kinds of sexual misconduct among severely and profoundly retarded persons, such as disrobing, may be etiologically distinct from the same behavior in nonretarded populations.

Treatment Research

Whatever the actual prevalence of sexual offenses among mentally retarded populations, sexual misconduct appears to account for a large proportion of the socially disapproved behavior that results in the removal of mentally retarded persons from society. Effective treatment for such offenders is critical. Service providers have recognized the need for specialized interventions for mentally retarded offenders, but research in this area is virtually nonexistent. Small-scale research and development efforts should design and pilot innovative strategies for treating mentally retarded offenders. Although mentally retarded persons learn slowly, they may be more responsive to treatment than some nonretarded offenders. Across a wide range of skill areas, mentally retarded persons continue to push back the threshold of expected abilities, showing that they are amenable to interventions once judged beyond the reach of persons of lower intellect (Scibak, 1983; Schinke & Olson, 1982; Wodarski & Bagarozzi, 1979). Researchers should collaborate with practitioners who are exploring ways of adapting standard sexual offender treatments for use with mentally retarded populations. A lack of sexual knowledge and experience may contribute to sex offenses by mentally retarded persons, and approaches that attempt to remedy these deficits in the context of sexual offender treatment should also be tested (Foxx, McMorrow, Storey, & Rogers, 1984; Murphy, Coleman, & Haynes, 1983).

Ethical Issues

Research on mentally retarded sex offenders is fraught with risks. Persons who are mentally retarded, often youthful, and sometimes confined in penal, psychiatric, or residential institutions, are vulnerable. Investigators who study mentally retarded populations, to a far greater extent than practitioners, must demonstrate that subjects' rights to informed consent are not violated (Gilchrist & Schinke, in press; Noonan & Bickel, 1981). Because sexual behavior itself is considered a private matter, research on sexuality raises a host of ethical dilemmas. No less troublesome are the risks that offenders pose to society.

Ethical and legal issues arise when researchers attempt new treatments, even when conventional intervention strategies have marginal or unknown efficacy. Given these risks and attendant procedural complexities, it is perhaps not surprising that little research has been done with mentally retarded sexual offenders. Along with the potential for abuse of human subjects, research review panels should consider the ultimate consequences to society and subject populations when protocols for research on human subjects serve to discourage entire areas of needed research.

CONCLUSION

The sexuality of mentally retarded persons remains a controversial and often misunderstood societal concern. History has shown that when knowledge about the capabilities and characteristics of persons with mental retardation is limited, society has been all too willing to form preconceived notions about the risks posed by retarded populations. Although the image of the "oversexed" mentally retarded person has not been completely eliminated, parents, professionals, and the public have become more accepting of the sexuality of mentally handicapped persons.

Unfortunately, knowledge about the relationship between mental retardation and sexual assault remains limited, and affords few ready answers for policy makers, practitioners, or advocates. Until carefully conducted studies provide better data, it is probably safe to conclude that sexual behavior, like other areas of social adaptation, remains potentially problematic for mentally retarded persons. Unquestionably, sexual offenses result in the institutionalization of mentally handicapped persons. Treatment providers have recognized that interventions must be adapted for mentally retarded offenders, and some have articulated strategies for such persons.

Theory-driven and empirically derived interventions, however, await testing in controlled program evaluations with mentally retarded sex offenders. Now is the time for creative practitioners and applied researchers to collaborate in conducting studies of treatment outcomes. Perhaps the present review and critical assessment of evidence, issues, and research needs will encourage other social work investigators to address gaps in the scientific evaluation and treatment of mentally retarded sex offenders.

REFERENCES

Abel, G. G., Rouleau, J., & Cunningham-Rathner, J. (in press). Sexually aggressive behavior. In W. Curran, A. L. McGarry, & S. A. Shah (Eds.), *Modern legal psychiatry and psychology*. Philadelphia: F. A. Davis.

Becker, J. V., Kaplan, M. S., Cunningham-Rathner, J., & Kavoussi, R. (1986). Characteristics of adolescent incest sexual perpetrators: Preliminary findings. *Journal of Family Violence, 1*(1), 13-26.

Berlin, F. S. (1983). Sex offenders: A biomedical perspective and a status report on biomedical treatment. In J. G. Greer & I. R. Stuart (Eds.), *The sexual aggressor: Current perspectives on treatment* (pp. 83-123). New York: Van Nostrand.

Brantlinger, E. (1983). Measuring variation and change in attitudes of residential care staff toward the sexuality of mentally retarded persons. *Mental Retardation, 21*(1), 17-22.

Craft, A., & Craft, M. (1981). Sexuality and mental handicap: A review. *British Journal of Psychiatry, 139*, 494-505.

de la Cruz, F. F., & La Veck, G. D. (1973). *Human sexuality and the mentally retarded*. New York: Brunner/Mazel.

Edgerton, R. B., & Dingman, H. (1964). Good reasons for bad supervision: Dating in a hospital for mentally retarded. *Psychiatric Quarterly Supplement Part 2*, 221-223.

Edmonson, B., McCombs, K., & Wish, J. (1979). What retarded adults believe about sex. *American Journal of Mental Deficiency, 84*(1), 11-18.

Ellis, A. (1970). The essence of rational psychotherapy: A comprehensive approach to treatment. New York: Institute for Rational Living.

Fehrenbach, P. A., Smith, W., Monastersky, C., & Deisher, R. W. (1986).

Adolescent sexual offenders: Offender and offense characteristics. *American Journal of Orthopsychiatry, 56*(2), 225-233.

Floor, L., Baxter, D., Rosen, M., & Zisfein, L. (1975). A survey of marriages among previously institutionalized retardates. *Mental Retardation, 13*, 33-37.

Foxx, R. M., McMorrow, M. J., Storey, K., & Rogers, B. M. (1984). Teaching social/sexual skills to mentally retarded adults. *American Journal of Mental Deficiency, 89*(1), 9-15.

Gilchrist, L. D., & Schinke, S. P. (in press). Ethics. In R. M. Grinnell, Jr. (Ed.), *Social work research and evaluation* (3rd ed.). Itasca, IL: F. E. Peacock.

Gochros, H. L., & Gochros, J. S. (1977). *The sexually oppressed.* New York: Association Press.

Gross, G. (1985). *Activities of the developmental disabilities adult offender project.* (Annual report September 6, 1983-September 30, 1984). Olympia, WA: Washington State Developmental Disabilities Planning Council.

Haskins, J. R., & Friel, C. B. (1972). *Strategies for the care and treatment of the mentally retarded,* Project CAMIO, Vol. 1.

Haywood, H. C. (1981). Reducing social vulnerability is the challenge of the eighties. *Mental Retardation, 19*, 190-195.

Heshusius, L. (1982). Sexuality, intimacy, and persons we label mentally retarded: What they think—what we think. *Mental Retardation, 20*(4), 164-168.

Jackson, I. F. (1984). *A preliminary survey of adolescent sex offenses in New York: Remedies and recommendations.* Syracuse, NY: Safer Society Press.

Johnson, P. R. (1984). Community-based sexuality programs for developmentally handicapped adults. In J. M. Berg (Ed.), *Perspectives and progress in mental retardation: Vol. 1. Social, psychological, and educational aspects.* Baltimore: University Park Press.

Knopp, F. H. (1984). *Retraining adult sexual offenders: Methods and models.* Syracuse, NY: Safer Society Press.

Knopp, F. H., Rosenberg, J., & Stevenson, W. (1986). *Report on nationwide survey of juvenile and adult sex-offender treatment programs and providers.* Syracuse, NY: Safer Society Press.

Landesman-Dwyer, S., & Sulzbacher, F. M. (1981). Residential placement and adaptation of severely and profoundly retarded individuals. In R. H. Bruininks, C. E. Meyers, B. B. Sigford, & K. C. Lakin (Eds.), *Deinstitutionalization and community adjustment of mentally retarded people* (Monograph no. 4). Washington, DC: American Association on Mental Deficiency.

Lanyon, R. I. (1986). Theory and treatment in child molestation. *Journal of Consulting and Clinical Psychology, 54*(2), 176-182.

Murphy, W. D., Coleman, E. M., & Abel, G. G. (1983). Human sexuality in the mentally retarded. In J. L. Matson & F. Andrasik (Eds.), *Treatment issues and innovations in mental retardation* (pp. 581-643). New York: Plenum Press.

Murphy, W. D., Coleman, E. M., & Haynes, M. R. (1983). Treatment and evaluation issues with the mentally retarded sex offender. In J. G. Greer & I. R. Stuart (Eds.), *The sexual aggressor: Current perspectives on treatment* (pp. 22-41). New York: Van Nostrand.

Noonan, M. J., & Bickel, W. K. (1981). The ethics of experimental design. *Mental Retardation, 19*(6), 271-274.

Reed, S. C., & Anderson, V. E. (1973). Effects of changing sexuality on the gene pool. In F. F. de la Cruz & G. D. La Veck (Eds.), *Human sexuality and the mentally retarded*. New York: Brunner/Mazel.

Robinson, N. M., & Robinson, H. B. (1976). *The mentally retarded child* (2nd ed.). New York: McGraw-Hill.

Santamour, M. B., & West, B. (1979). A clinical and practical discussion of retardation and criminal behavior. In *Retardation and criminal justice: A training manual for criminal justice personnel*. President's Committee on Mental Retardation.

Schilling, R. F., & Schinke, S. P. (1984). Maltreatment and mental retardation. In J. M. Berg (Ed.), *Perspectives and progress in mental retardation: Vol. 1. Social, psychological, and educational aspects* (pp. 11-22). Baltimore: University Park Press.

Schilling, R. F., Schinke, S. P., Blythe, B. J., & Barth, R. P. (1982). Child maltreatment and mentally retarded parents: Is there a relationship? *Mental Retardation, 20,* 201-209.

Schinke, S. P., & Olson, D. G. (1982). Home-based remediation of subacute sclerosing panencephalitis. *Education and Treatment of Children, 5,* 261-269.

Scibak, J. W. (1983). Behavioral treatment. In J. L. Matson & J. A. Mulick (Eds.), *Handbook of mental retardation* (pp. 339-350). New York: Pergamon Press.

Shoor, M., Speed, M. H., & Bartelt, C. (1966). Syndrome of the adolescent child molester. *American Journal of Psychiatry, 122,* 783-789.

Timmers, R. L., DuCharme, P., & Jacob, G. (1981). Sexual knowledge, attitudes and behaviors of developmentally disabled adults living in a normalized apartment setting. *Sexuality and Disability, 4*(1), 27-39.

Wodarski, J. S., & Bagarozzi, D. A. (1979). *Behavioral social work*. New York: Human Sciences Press.

Yochelson, S., & Samenow, S. E. (1977). *The criminal personality*, Vols. 1 & 2. New York: Jason Aronson.

Zetlin, A. G., & Turner, J. L. (1985). Transition from adolescence to adulthood: Perspectives of mentally retarded individuals and their families. *American Journal of Mental Deficiency, 89*(6), 570-579.

Treatment of Sexual Offenders in a Community Mental Health Center: An Evaluation

Daniel L. Whitaker
John S. Wodarski

SUMMARY. The manuscript reviews the literature concerning sexual offenders. Specific topics discussed are characteristics of the sexual offender, dangerousness, cultural influences, and typologies of sexual crimes. A comprehensive treatment program utilized with nonviolent sexual offenders is elaborated. Outcome measures used to evaluate the program are presented. A discussion of the implications of the study for the field of social work concludes the manuscript.

"The ubiquity of sex in the mind of people is nowhere more apparent than in the variety of devices that have been contrived to limit its free expression" (Kozol, Cohen, & Garofalo, 1976). Americans, although permissive in some areas of behavior such as freedom of speech and business enterprise, are more restrictive than most other western societies in laws about sex (Slovenko, 1965). At one time or another almost every type of interpersonal sexual activity has been condemned. Societies have labeled masturbation, premarital sex, oral-genital relations, and homosexual activity as criminal (Ford & Beach, 1951). There are many sexual acts that are still punishable in the United States according to the law. As a matter of

Preparation of this manuscript was facilitated by a special projects grant funded through the Office of the Vice-President for Research, University of Georgia Research Foundation; general operating budget, University of Georgia School of Social Work; an award by the National Institute of Mental Health, Social Work Education Branch MH13753 and MH17208.

fact, one expert has estimated that 9 out of every 10 persons in the United States is "technically a sex criminal" (Kinsey, Pomeroy, & Martin, 1948). Many of the condemned sexual practices, however, are regarded by the general population as either a private matter or quite acceptable.

An extensive revision of the laws regulating sex has been proposed, on the grounds that "imposing long prison terms for behavior which is widely practiced by the general public is neither good sense or good law" (Kling, 1965). This has occurred in conjunction with the clamor for the imposition of longer prison sentences for sex crimes. Public reaction to a particularly heinous or despicable crime or series of sexual offenses reported in the media often creates political pressure upon legislatures to do something. Legislators frequently react by calling for the imposition of longer prison sentences for sexual crimes. In one instance they demanded the death penalty for child molestation (Atlanta Journal Staff, 1984). The question of how society can protect itself from criminal acts in a humane way and without creating more problems remains unanswered.

For centuries, sexual behavior that violates the accepted societal norms has been a matter for social control and, in civilized societies, for legal control through criminal sanction (Editor, *Georgia Law Review*, 1969). Sodom and Gomorrah supposedly were destroyed to control aberrant sexual behavior. The rationale for attempting to control sexual behavior is often based on the perceived need to channel sexual drive into forms of conduct leading to procreation, production of stable family units, protection and socialization of the young, and thereby perpetuation of the society (Kling, 1965). Some scholars assert that social control is necessary because of the antisocial force inherent in the competitive nature of the sex drive (Davis & Sines, 1971).

Social control is brought about by decreeing that certain behaviors are deviant or illegal. Most societies select certain sexual behaviors as acceptable and often proscribe all others (Ford & Beach, 1951). An individual who has violated one of the "sex laws" is known as a "sex offender."

For social work practice, the literature on methods of treating the sexual offender is limited. Moreover, virtually no research has been carried out to evaluate the treatment approaches proposed. This manuscript reviews relevant literature, presents data on the evaluation of a specific treatment approach, and briefly discusses the implications of the approach for practice.

CHARACTERISTICS OF THE SEX OFFENDER

The most detailed and comprehensive studies of sex offenders are those of Albert Ellis and Ralph Brancale (1956) at the New Jersey Diagnostic Center and Radzenowicz (1968) at Cambridge University. Both studies were conducted in the early 1950s. A third well-known study of sex offenders is that of Gebhard, Gagnon, Pomeroy, and Christianson (1965) of the Kinsey Sex Institute. Gebhard et al. primarily studied incarcerated sex offenders. Ellis and Brancale used data from 300 men convicted of a sex crime in New Jersey in 1949-1950. These three studies, and the majority of the other descriptive studies as well, show two common themes: that most sex offenders are "mild and submissive" and that, of the various types of criminals, they are the least likely to repeat.

Exhibitionists make up the largest group of sex offenders, implicated in about 30% of all sex offenses (Henninger, 1941). Exhibitionists are usually married men. Married or formerly married men made up 64% of the population in the Gebhard study, 62% in the Radzenowicz study, and a high of 79% in a study reported of an outpatient population in Toronto (Mohr, Turner, & Jerry, 1964). Although the marriage rate was high, the marriages were not very fruitful. In the Kinsey Institute study of 288 exhibitionists, where the average age of the offenders was 35, there were only 10 children among 14 couples. In the Radzenowicz study, a high percentage of the marriages produced only one child. There was a smaller percentage of marriages among rapists (48%) and an even smaller percentage among homosexual offenders (23%).

Kopp (1962) reports that many sex offenders feel dominated by women. Foobert, Bartelme, and Jones (1958) used the MMPI to compare 160 non-sex-offender inmates at San Quentin Prison with 120 child molesters. An item analysis indicated that child molesters were strongly religious, were dissatisfied sexually, felt inadequate in their interpersonal relations, and were very sensitive to others' evaluations.

Panton (1958) reports the ability to separate sex offenders from other crime classification groups through use of the MMPI. Differences among the profiles of rapists of adults, rapists of children, and nonviolent molesters of female children were found (Panton, 1978). Anderson, Kunce, and Brice (1979) report three personality types for sex offenders. An analysis of MMPI profiles of 92 sex offenders revealed that 88 were masculinity-femininity, schizophrenia (Mf, Sc); psychopathic deviant, hypomania (Pd, Hy); or depression, psychopathic deviant (D, Pd) profile types.

Ellis and Brancale (1956) found a higher incidence of pathology among exhibitionists. Six percent were diagnosed as psychopathic personality while 3.4% were found to be mentally deficient. The expected percentage of mentally deficient in the general population is 2.2%. Arieff and Rotman (1942) reported 26% of their sample to be compulsive neurotics; 14% were mentally retarded. Mohr et al. (1964) found a normal IQ distribution in WAIS scores in their outpatient population but noted a phenomenon of educational underachievement. In their population, only 1 in 54 reached university level. They noted that the peak period of onset of exhibitionist symptoms in the mid-teens coincided with the average age of school dropout. They noted that this most likely contributed to the low educational level.

In a study of 16- to 19-year-old male sex offenders, Longo (1982) found that many had begun to learn about sex before they reached puberty and had sexual experiences with adults generally eight years older than themselves. They concluded that sex offenders do not have normal psychosexual histories.

Studies of characteristics of sex offenders indicate a heterogeneous grouping. The diversity is more apparent than any similarities. If, however, sex offenders are separated into two groups according to the amount of violence involved, common themes surface. Nonviolent sex offenders are less aggressive and more withdrawn and are more likely to recidivate (Greane, 1977). Violent offenders, on the other hand, are less likely to repeat their offenses but are more likely to be hostile. They also abuse alcohol and hate or resist authority (Ellis & Brancale, 1956). Treatment procedures would more likely be successful with separate programs for the two groups.

DANGEROUSNESS AND THE SEX OFFENDER

Americans are most concerned about crimes that affect their personal safety as they perceive it. Public perception of the probability that any individual will become a victim of violent crime is distorted by the news media's emphasis on criminal acts. The more gory and lurid the crime, the more attention is directed toward it (Winslow, 1973).

In establishing community-based treatment programs, the public's perception of the dangerousness of sex criminals must be considered (Abel, Blanchard, & Beecher, 1976). Public reaction to several violent sexual crimes in Massachusetts led to the creation of a quasi-medical diagnosis of "sexually dangerous person." Massachusetts law provides for an indeterminate sentence of one day to life if an individual is so adjudicated in a civil hearing (Kozol, Boucher, & Garofalo, 1972). Such laws, known as mentally disordered sex offender (MDSO) laws, have been controversial since the first of them was passed in Michigan in 1937. Conservatives charge that the indeterminate nature of MDSO laws allows sex offenders to be released too soon. Liberals charge that the MDSO laws are racially and economically discriminatory and are applied to persons for whom the presence of a serious mental disorder is questionable (Monahan & Davis, 1983).

As of January 1, 1980, 20 states had MDSO laws in effect, but a movement toward repeal has been noted (Dix, 1983). This movement is partially the result of a renewed interest in determinate sentencing but also represents a loss of faith in the efficacy of treatment programs and in the validity of the prediction of dangerousness. Tappan (1975), for example, has pointed out that indefinite commitment laws are morally justifiable only if there are accurate means to determine whether an offender is dangerous and if treatment is available.

Much of the social policy in the area of mental health and criminal justice is based on the assumption that psychiatrists, psychologists, and social workers can predict behavior (Monahan & Cummings, 1975). Is this assumption valid? If so, under what conditions? In discussing the issue of emergency-room assessments, Peske (1975) stated that "prediction of danger is not within medical competence" and should not be. He feels that physicians should not be expected "to act as agents of society" in making such decisions. Others have stated that "dangerousness" cannot be predicted in reference to discharges from mental hospitals (Dershowitz, 1971) or cases of suicide (Murphy, 1972).

Wenk, Robison, and Smith (1972) using elaborate case histories, current measures of mental and emotional functioning, and professional prognoses, were unable to develop a classification scheme for estimating potential for assault among parolees from California prisons. They discuss a number of methodological problems with attempts to predict violence, including the self-fulfilling nature of such labels. They conclude that predictions are not possible.

Schlesinger (1978) studied 39 predictors of violence from 12 different research studies. Using these predictors to assess the probability that 122 juveniles referred by judges would exhibit violent behavior, he was unable to substantiate their usefulness. The author states that "low base rate behaviors (such as dangerousness) cannot be predicted sufficiently to warrant their use in clinical practice" (Schlesinger, 1978).

Judgments about dangerousness are constantly being made, however, especially in the fields of criminal justice and mental health. What criteria can and should be used in making such judgments?

Kozel, Boucher, and Garofalo (1972) state that dangerousness can be reliably diagnosed and treated with accuracy. They report on a 10-year study of 592 males who had been adjudicated as dangerous sex offenders. Following treatment for an average period of 43 months, the offenders were no longer considered dangerous and were discharged. The recidivism rate was only 6%.

Their predictions of dangerousness were based on extensive clinical interviews by psychiatrists, psychologists, and social workers. They found that the description of the aggressor in action was the most useful predictor. Interviews with the victim by social workers were often compared with material obtained from the offender. Criteria were gathered in seven dimensions:

1. Did the offender use force and violence?
2. What is the offender's view of himself?
3. What is the offender's view of the victim?
4. What are the characteristics of the offender's relationships with others?
5. How does the offender view his future prospects?
6. What does he see as his relationship with the community?
7. What were his family relationships like? (Kozol, Boucher, & Garofalo, 1972)

Halleck (1971) also feels that dangerousness can be predicted only on the basis of clinical judgments. He states that no single factor "is a necessary or sufficient predictor."

Although the research seems to show no clear-cut syndrome, several gross predictors of dangerousness seem appropriate. The first predictor is a history of violence (Winslow, 1973). The Bridgewater group, for instance, flatly state that "no one can predict dangerous behavior in an individual with no history of dangerous acting out" (Kozol, Boucher, & Garofalo, 1972). A second predictor, called the "essence of dangerousness," is a lack of feeling or concern for others. When combined with anger, this often leads to violent behaviors (Rappaport, 1967).

Until dangerousness can be predicted reliably, it should be assumed that the best way to ensure safe treatment in a community mental health center is to make support and control available in the community while treatment is being instituted (Cohen, Groth, & Siegal, 1978).

CULTURAL INFLUENCES

Most cultures have developed elaborate social patterns of behavior surrounding genital aspects of sex (Barlow & Winze, 1980). Alfred Kinsey and his colleagues (1948) have pointed out that it has been criminal to encourage masturbation in some legal jurisdictions of the United States. That is, to teach, counsel, or advise another to masturbate is illegal. They have also pointed out a class distinction in the social acceptance of the practice.

Certain anthropologists have asserted that the sex drive is so competitive and "instinctively anarchic" that it is necessary in any society to set up norms for the regulation of sexual conduct (Davis, 1971). Some experts believe that all animals are sexually violent and that violent behavior during foreplay has an important function (Ford & Beach, 1951). This observation may explain in part the finding in one study that 12 to 16% of heterosexual aggressors believed that force and violence were a necessary part of obtaining sexual goals (Gebhard, Gagnon, Pomeroy, & Christianson, 1965). It is more plausible, however, to ascribe such behavior to a culture or subculture of violence rather than to biological factors (Groth & Burgess, 1977). Nonconsensual sex obtained by force is the most strongly condemned form of sexual activity, with the possible exception of incest (Ford & Beach, 1951).

In America many sexual feelings and behaviors have been equated with sin (Masters & Johnson, 1970). Manifestations of a need for sexual pleasure are apt to be denied, ignored, or thought of as shameful. Sex is often associated with painful consequences and discomfort, especially during the early years (Schimel, 1971).

The interaction between the child's developing sexual urges and the experiences of growing up in our sexually alienating society probably produces some measure of sexual conflict in all of us. Various studies have demonstrated that the individual's feeling of self-esteem relates to one's earliest experiences (Arieff & Rotman, 1942; MacDonald, 1973). It is those feelings that really determine the fate of the individual in all aspects of his being, including his sex life. Even in the first few months of life, an infant is extremely responsive to signs of favor or disfavor on the part of the caretakers (Schimel, 1971).

Most mothers of sex offenders are "prudish" (MacDonald, 1973). They are often sexually frigid themselves, with an attitude toward sex ranging from tolerance to outright contempt (Starr, 1965). Many sex offenders are therefore reared according to a rigid set of principles and taught that sex is disgusting and disgraceful.

As a result, they adapt to the negative consequences associated with the expression of sexuality with varying degrees of sexual alienation (Kaplan, 1974).

TYPOLOGIES OF SEX CRIMES

There is general agreement that sex offenders do not form a homogeneous group, and a number of typologies have been offered to classify them. Most have included some type of categorization by age (Glueck, 1965) or sex (Fitch, 1962; Frisbie & Dondis, 1965) of the victim or age (Gray & Mohr, 1965) of the offender, or both (Gebhard, Gagnon, Pomeroy, & Christianson, 1976). Otherschemes have been based on the psychiatric classification of the offender (West, 1965) and legal categories (MacNamara & Sagarin, 1977). Sex offenders have often been viewed as needing treatment for their inability to internalize sexual controls as opposed to punishment for an unwillingness to do so (Allen, 1969). None of the proposed typologies, however, address the need for a method of developing treatment programs that are suitable for community mental health centers.

There are three major classifications of sex offenders: the incest offender, the violent offender, and the social decency offender. The focus of treatment is necessarily different for each of these three types. Treatment for the incest offender focuses on family relationships and their modification. Incestual child molesters are a special case of situational offenders. They very seldom prefer children as sexual partners and are least likely to recidivate. Their offense is related to family dynamics and opportunism rather than inappropriate sexual preference. The procedure of treatment is the rebuilding of the marital dyad, reestablishing the mother/daughter relationship and reframing the cognitions and affective focus of the adult/child transactions. Following these separate actions, the family often can be successfully reconstituted.

The focus of treatment for the violent offender is to help him find an appropriate expression of anger and power. The violent offender often derives sexual pleasure from the use of unnecessary force and does not adequately comprehend the significance of responses to the force. He may also use force when he loses control or feels he may use force to obtain his desires without concern for others (Brodsky & Hobart, 1978). The procedure for treatment is therefore to refocus aggression into appropriate socially acceptable channels, to teach appropriate means of expressing anger, and to aid the offender in obtaining a more stable control of his behavior.

The focus of treatment for the social decency offender is an appropriate expression of sexual feelings which are often immature (Christoffel, 1936). The procedure for treatment is to provide knowledge about sex, to increase the ability to communicate feelings, and to develop social skills. Social decency offenders often are deficient in assertion skills and need training in these as well.

The following treatment program was designed and implemented for social decency offenders, those convicted of nonviolent crimes that did not directly involve family members. Participants were expected to develop new means of expressing sexual feelings; to communicate their needs, wants, and desires without guilt; and to exhibit increased personal feelings of self-esteem. The purpose of this investigation was to study the effects of participation in a multifocused, time-limited treatment group on certainty of self-perception, self-acceptance, perception of personal worth, satisfaction with social interactions, assertiveness, acceptance as a family member, and self-esteem of male sex offenders.

TREATMENT PROGRAM AND SETTING

The treatment group participated in 16 weekly sessions of one and one-half hours each. An additional group session was held before the beginning of treatment and another after the completion of treatment for data collection. The treatment group was structured in nature. The content included (1) structured exercises, (2) role play, (3) demonstrations, and (4) small-group discussions using both didactic and experiential methods. Table 1 provides an outline of each session's treatment objectives.

The treatment sessions were held at and were part of the overall program of the Cobb-Douglas Community Mental Health Center, which serves two counties located in metropolitan Atlanta. Approximately 390,000 persons reside in the two-county area. The facility is centrally located and is attached to a general hospital.

There were three group leaders, one female and two males. The female therapist was an MSW social worker. One of the male therapists was an MEd counselor; the other an MSW graduate student. The treatment foci were sex awareness, communication/social skills, and assertion skills. Each group leader chose the treatment focus he or she was most interested in and was responsible for that area at each session. The sex awareness focus was the responsibility of the female therapist, by her choice. Time allotments for the primary areas varied for each session but were approximately equal over all.

GROUP MEMBERS

The members of the group were referred by probation officers and by therapists in the Center. Criteria for referral to the group were that the person should:

1. Be at least 18 years of age,
2. Be safe to be "at large,"
3. Not be a substance abuser,
4. Have no organic condition which might hinder relearning,
5. Have normal intelligence,
6. Have no thought disorder,
7. Be amenable to treatment.

Persons referred were interviewed by one of the three therapists, and a complete psychosocial and a mental status examination were done. After each group member was seen separately by a staff psychiatrist, a diagnosis was assigned. Nine men were interviewed for the group; seven of these participated. One person dropped out when pending charges were dropped. Another was not included due to work scheduling problems.

The Minnesota Multiphasic Personality Inventory (MMPI), the Tennessee Self Concept Scale (TSCS), and a Rathus Assertiveness Schedule (RAS) were administered to each group member before

Table 1

Session Outlines

Session	Sexual Awareness	Communication-Social Skills	Assertiveness	General
Introduction				Program philosophy
1			Introduce group members	Program structure and method
2	Slang terms	Interpersonal communication principles	Define "Assertion"	
3	Slang terms	Analyzing interpersonal transactions	Deep muscle relaxation, covert desensitization	
4	Slang terms	Transactional analysis	Assertion myths	
5	Sexual questions	Cross transactions	SUDS	
6	Personal sexual concerns	Strokes	Develop assertion goals	
7	Personal sexual concerns	Bumper sticker communications	Assertion training diary	
8	Sexual questions	Games analysis	Finalize assertion goals	
9	Homosexual myths	Drama triangle	Assertive behavior role play	

Table 1 (continued)

Session Outlines

Session	Sexual Awareness	Communication-Social Skills	Assertiveness	General
10	Personal sexual responses	Script analysis	Assertion role play	
11	"Fishbowl"			
12	Process "Fishbowl"	Life positions	Assertion skills practice	
13	Discuss sex offense			Review treatment goals
14		Utilize skills in group	Role play work situations	
15	Public sexual attitudes	Utilize skills in group		
16		Utilize skills in group		Closure
Final		Obtain feedback from group	Evaluation of goals	Obtain post-treatment data

and at the end of the treatment period. Scores from the tests were used as outcome measures.

The MMPI is a standard screening device often used in the detection of psychopathology. RAS purports to measure changes in assertion. The various sub-scales of the TSCS were used to measure selected facets of self-perception in which changes were predicted.

Table 2 presents the types of sex offenders in the group by sex offense. Individuals in the group ranged in age from 18 to 48 years of age with an average age of 31 years. Two of the members were divorced. Four of the members had never married. All four of the single men still lived at home with their parents. Only one member of the group had fathered a child, and he had not had contact with the child in more than three years.

DESIGN

The experimental design used was a One Group Pretest-Posttest Design. This design contains measures for an aggregate of individuals at two time periods, making it possible to employ statistical procedures (Tripodi, 1983). Although not controlling for some alternative explanations for change, the design does provide a first approximation of cause-effect knowledge.

RESULTS

The means, standard deviations, and levels of significance of the outcome variables are recorded in Table 3. Significant differences were found between the pretreatment and posttreatment means of three of the eight dependent variables: self-satisfaction, family interaction, and certainty. In addition, differences between the means for three of the five remaining dependent variables were found to be in the predicted direction. It should be noted that although significant changes were made in some areas, it was not the judgment of the therapists that no further treatment was needed. A continuing group concentrating on social interaction skills and the development of personal awareness was recommended to probation officers.

Table 2

Types of Sex Offenders in Group by Offense

	Number	Percent
Sodomy	1	14.3
Obscene Phone Caller	2	28.5
Indecent Exposure	3	42.8
Voyeur	1	14.3
TOTAL	7	100.0

COLLATERAL FINDINGS

Collateral findings are those findings which, although serving to support or corroborate primary findings, are of a secondary nature. The male version of the "Sex Concerns Checklist" of the sex education package *About Your Sexuality* by Deryck Calderwood (1983) was given to group members as part of the third group session. The purpose of the Sex Concerns Checklist was to gather information useful in determining appropriate directions for the sex education modules. Responses indicated group members had a number of concerns about individual sexuality which were indicative of naiveté. These concerns included being able to have intercourse correctly, the desire to see the nude body of a female, and to look at or own sexually exciting pictures or books. Discussions by the members indicated gross misunderstandings of female rights and sexuality which contributes to social anxiety and disturbed social interactions (Calderwood, 1983). These findings indicate a strong need for sexual awareness components to be included in any treatment programs for sex offenders.

IMPLICATIONS

One task of the social work profession is to continue to develop preventive roles (Wodarski, 1981). The data obtained in this study indicate a number of useful tasks for social workers which might aid in the reduction of sex offenses through preventive actions. Sex

Table 3

Means, Standard Deviations and Levels of Significance of the Outcome Variables

Variables	Means		Standard Deviations		Levels of Significance
	Pre-Treatment	Post-Treatment	Pre-Treatment	Post-Treatment	
Self-esteem	261.14	268.71	19.4	18.4	.10
Self-satisfaction	89.71	95.14	10.7	7.5	.04*
Sexuality	55.71	54.57	4.9	5.2	.50
Family Interaction	55.43	58.00	6.4	5.9	.01
Personal Worth	46.86	50.30	2.4	4.4	.07
Social Interaction	53.86	52.70	3.8	5.8	.53
Certainty	96.43	79.86	19.5	8.9	.01
Assertiveness	7.43	23.57	11.3	23.0	.06

offenders show significant naiveté and gross misconceptions about female sexuality. They also lack social and communication skills. They have many questions and doubts about their individual sexuality. Often it is these deficiencies that bring them to the attention of the criminal justice system. Sex education programs and social/communication skills groups would serve to prevent deviant expression of sexual feelings. This implies, of course, some mechanism for identifying such persons before the commission of an offense.

The findings of this study also indicate that one group of sex offenders can make significant changes in self-perception as part of an outpatient treatment program in a community mental health center. This is possible at a much lower cost and less severe disruption to family life as compared to incarceration. Treatment in the community further serves to maintain the offender as a contributing member.

Without adequate professional preparation, social workers will continue to have difficulty participating in sex offense prevention and treatment programs. Presently, reports of sexual abuse of children at home and in day-care facilities appear daily in the media. Few social workers receive adequate training to prepare them for the tasks they face in investigating, treating, and preventing these events. This study represents a first step toward development and evaluation of a treatment program based on current empirical knowledge.

REFERENCES

Abel, G. G., Blanchard, E. B., & Beecher, J. V. (1976). An integrated treatment program for rapists. In R. Rada (Ed.), *Clinical aspects of the rapist*. New York: Gruve & Stratton.

Allen, C. (1969). *A textbook of psychosocial disorders*. New York: Oxford University Press.

Anderson, W. P., Kunce, J. T., & Brice, R. (1979). Sex offenders: Three personality types. *Journal of Clinical Psychology, 35*(3), 671-676.

Arieff, A. J., & Rotman, D. B. (1942). One hundred cases of indecent exposure. *Journal of Nervous and Mental Disorders, 96*, 523.

Atlanta Journal Staff. (1984, February 2). Molestation penalty increased by house. *Atlanta Journal.*

Barlow, D. H., & Winze, J. P. (1980). Treatment of sexual deviations. In S.

Leiblum & L. Pervin (Eds.), *Principles and practice of sex therapy.* New York: Guilford Press.

Brodsky, S. L., & Hobart, S. C. (1978). Blame models and assailant research. *Criminal Justice and Behavior, 5*(4), 319-388.

Calderwood, D. (1983). *About your sexuality.* Boston: Beacon Press.

Christoffel, H. (1936). Exhibitionism and exhibitionists. *International Journal of Psychoanalysis, 17*, 321.

Cohen, M., Groth, N., & Siegal, R. (1978, January). The clinical prediction of dangerousness. *Crime and Delinquency*, pp. 28-39.

Cohen, M. L., Seghorn, T., & Calmas, P. (1969). Sociometric study of the sex offender. *Journal of Abnormal Psychology, 74*, 249-255.

Davis, K. (1971). Sexual behavior. In R. Merton & R. Nisbut (Eds.), *Contemporary social problems.* New York: Harcourt Brace.

Davis, K., & Sines, J. (1971). An antisocial behavioral pattern associated with a specific MMPI profile. *Journal of Consulting and Clinical Psychology, 36*, 229-234.

Dershowitz, A. M. (1971). The law of dangerousness: Some fictions about predictions. *Journal of Legal Education, 23*(1), 24-47.

Dix, G. E. (1983). Special dispositional alternatives for abnormal offenders. In *Mentally disordered offenders.* New York: Plenum Press.

Editor. (1969). Pedophilia, exhibitionism and voyeurism: Legal problems in the deviant society. *Georgia Law Review, 4*, 149-163.

Ellis, A., & Brancale, R. (1956). *The psychology of sex offenders.* Springfield, IL: Charles C Thomas.

Fitch, J. H. (1962). Men convicted of sexual offenses against children. *British Journal of Criminology, 3*, 18-37.

Foobert, S., Bartelme, K., & Jones, E. (1958). Some factors related to pedophilia. *International Journal of Social Psychiatry, 4*, 272-279.

Ford, C. S., & Beach, F. A. (1951). *Patterns of sexual behavior.* New York: Harper.

Frisbie, L. V., & Dondis, E. H. (1965). Recidivism among treated sex offenders. *California Mental Health Research Monograph, 5*, 1 + .

Gebhard, P. H., Gagnon, J. H., Pomeroy, W. B., & Christianson, C. V. (1965). *Sex offenders: An analysis of types.* New York: Harper & Row.

Gebhard, P. H., Gagnon, J. H., Pomeroy, W. B., & Christianson, C. V. (1976). Sex offenders: An analysis of types. In M. Weinberg (Ed.), *Sex research studies from the Kinsey Institute.* New York: Oxford University Press.

Glueck, B. C., Jr., (1965). Pedophilia. In R. Slovenko (Ed.), *Sexual behavior and the law.* Springfield, IL: Charles C Thomas.

Gray, K. G., & Mohr, J. W. (1965). Follow-up of male sexual offenders. In R. Slovenko (Ed.), *Sexual behaviors and the law.* Springfield, IL: Charles C Thomas.

Greane, R. S. (1977). Contemporary dilemmas in personality assessment illustrated in a diagnostic case study. *Perceptual and Motor Skills, 44*(3), 967-973.

Groth, A. N., & Burgess, A. W. (1977). Rape: A sexual deviation. *American Journal of Orthopsychiatry, 97*(3), 400-406.

Halleck, S. (1971). *Psychiatry and the dilemmas of crime.* Berkeley: University of California Press.

Henninger, J. M. (1941). Exhibitionism. *Journal of Criminal Psychopathology, 2,* 357.

Kaplan, H. S. (1974). *The new sex therapy.* New York: Brunner/Mazel.

Kinsey, A. C., Pomeroy, W. B., & Martin, C. E. (1948). *Sexual behavior in the human male.* Philadelphia: Saunders.

Kling, S. G. *Sexual behavior and the law.* (1965). New York: Random House.

Kopp, S. B. (1962). The character structure of sex offenders. *American Journal of Psychotherapy, 16,* 64.

Kozol, H., Boucher, R., & Garofalo, R. (1972). The diagnosis and treatment of dangerousness. *Crime and Delinquency, 18,* 371-392.

Kozol, H., Cohen, M. I., & Garofalo, R. (1976). The criminally dangerous sex offender. *New England Journal of Medicine, 275*(29), 79-84.

Longo, R. E. (1982). Sexual learning and experience among adolescent sexual offenders. *International Journal of Offender Therapy and Comparative Criminology, 26*(3), 235-241.

MacDonald, J. M. (1973). *Indecent exposure.* Springfield, IL: Charles C Thomas.

MacNamara, D. E. J., & Sagarin, E. (1977). *Sex crime and the law.* New York: MacMillan.

Masters, W. H., & Johnson, V. E. (1970). *The pleasure bond.* New York: Benton Books.

Mohr, J. W., Turner, R. E., & Jerry, M. B. (1964). *Pedophilia and exhibitionism.* Toronto: University of Toronto Press.

Monahan, J., & Cummings, L. (1975, March). Social implications of the inability to predict violence. *Journal of Social Issues,* p. 3.

Monahan, J., & Davis, S. (1983). Mentally disordered sex offenders. In *Mentally disordered offenders.* New York: Plenum Press.

Murphy, G. E. (1972). Clinical identification of suicidal risk. *Archives of General Psychiatry, 27,* 356-359.

Panton, J. H. (1958). MMPI profile configurations among crime classification groups. *Journal of Clinical Psychology, 14,* 305-308.

Panton, J. H. (1978). Personality differences appearing between rapists of adults, rapists of children and non-violent sexual molesters of female children. *Research Communications in Psychology, Psychiatry and Behavior, 3*(4), 385-393.

Peske, M. A. (1975, August). Is dangerousness an issue for physicians in emergency commitments? *American Journal of Psychiatry,* p. 828.

Radzenowicz, L. (1968). *Sexual offenses: A report of the Cambridge Department of Criminal Science.* London: McMillan.

Rappaport, J. R. (Ed.). (1967). *The clinical evaluation of dangerousness of the mentally ill.* Springfield, IL: Charles C Thomas.

Schimel, J. L. (1971). Self-esteem and sex. *Sexual Behavior, 1*(4), 3-9.

Schlesinger, S. E. (1978, January). The prediction of dangerousness in juveniles: A replication. *Crime and Delinquency*, pp. 40-48.

Slovenko, R. (Ed.). (1965). *Sexual behavior and the law*. Springfield, IL: Charles C Thomas.

Starr, A. (1965). *Sexual deviation*. Baltimore: Penguin Books.

Tappan, P. W. (1975). Some myths about the sex offender. *Federal Probation, 6*, 7-12.

Tripodi, T. (1983). *Evaluative research for social workers*. Englewood Cliffs, NJ: Prentice-Hall.

Wenk, E. A., Robison, J. O., & Smith, G. W. (1972). Can violence be predicted? *Crime and Delinquency*, pp. 393-402.

West, D. J. (1965). Clinical types among sexual offenders. In R. Slovenko (Ed.), *Sexual behavior and the law*. Springfield, IL: Charles C Thomas.

Winslow, R. (Ed.). (1973). *Crime in a free society*. Encino, CA: Dickerson.

Wodarski, J. S. (1981). *The role of research in clinical practice*. Baltimore: University Park Press.

Incest Family Dynamics:
Family Members' Perceptions
Before and After Therapy

Inger J. Sagatun
Louise Prince

SUMMARY. A self-administered questionnaire study in a self-help group for incest families focused on individual family members' perceptions of their interrelationships before and after participation in therapy. The results show that perceptions of the same relationships varied greatly among family members. Before therapy, the father-daughter relationship received the most divergent ratings, with fathers rating it as extremely good and daughters as extremely bad. The mother-daughter relationship was seen as the most neutral by all family members. After therapy, while the parents improved their perceptions of family relations, daughters (victims) continued to rate them as bad. It is suggested that the emphasis on teaching victims to externalize the blame in order to diminish unjust guilt and shame in effect means shifting the blame to the father (the offender), which again serves to maintain stressful family relations for the daughters in these families. The clinical implications of this dilemma are discussed.

This paper looks at incest family members' perceptions of their family relationships before and after therapy and explores how these perceptions are affected by court-ordered participation in therapy programs.

Most discussions of incest suggest that it occurs in highly dis-

The authors wish to thank the members of Parents United for their participation in this research. This study was supported by a grant from the University of California, Riverside, to the first author. An earlier version of this paper was presented at the American Sociological Association Meetings in Washington DC, 1985.

69

turbed or in character-disordered families (e.g., Anderson & Shafer, 1979; Raphling, Carpenter, & Davis, 1967). Some have described the mother-daughter relationship as particularly estranged (Herman & Hirschman, 1977; Kaufman, Peck, & Tagiuri, 1954), while others have focused on the traumatic father-daughter relationship (Browning & Boatman, 1977). The parental relationship is generally assumed to be poor, although this is seldom specifically studied. None of the studies focuses on the problems of conflicting perceptions of family relationships held by the various family members. We suggest that a disturbing characteristic of incest families is the failure to agree on the nature of family relationships. Often, perhaps because of poor communication skills, incest family members have very different perceptions of the value and strength of their interpersonal relations. This paper therefore looks at how all three groups in father-daughter incest families (father, daughters, and mothers) view the father-daughter, the mother-daughter, and the father-mother relationship, both before and after therapeutic intervention.

According to Herman and Hirschman (1977), the most striking fact in incest families is the almost uniform estrangement of the mother and daughter, an estrangement that often precedes the occurrence of overt incest. Over half of the mothers in their studies were incapacitated either physically or psychologically, and their daughters were obliged to take over the household duties. Previous studies of incestuous families also document the disturbance of the mother-father relationship as a constant finding. Kaufman, Peck, and Tagiuri (1954) focused on the family situation in which the traditional mother-daughter roles were reversed. The mother often turned over to the daughter much of the household responsibilities, and the mother's own inability to relate sexually to her husband contributed to creating a situation where father and daughter found themselves together because of the mother's abandonment. The child was left neglected and vulnerable. According to Lustig et al. (1966), a wife will often, consciously or unconsciously, sanction the incestual relationship between father and daughter. She can be a silent partner in initiating and sustaining the incestuous relationship. Weiss et al. (1955) argued that the daughter's deprivation by and resentment of her mother is the basic conflict underlying the sexual trauma in incest families. As a response to the mother's lack of interest, the father often begins to single out the oldest daughter both to fill a maternal family role and to participate in a secret sexual relationship. As that daughter advances into adolescence and becomes more rebellious, the fathers may move on to a younger sister.

When the daughter and the mother do not get along, the daughter may seek an affectionate relationship with the father. According to Koch (1980) sexuality and affection may merge, and the father may justify the sexual relationship with the daughter as being an expression of love. Gentry (1978) writes that contrary to popular opinion, there is generally much genuine caring and affection in incestuous families. Spencer (1978) writes of early father-daughter incest as the "courting period" where the father-daughter relationship is sensed by the rest of the family as a "special" relationship. She argues that the sexual activity often does not involve actual penetration until the child has become conditioned to the father's advances, and in the process a real affection between father and daughter may have developed.

Others have given a less "positive" picture of this development. Browning and Boatman (1977) discuss how and why many daughters were *forced* to assume their mothers' role. They also note that many fathers in their study were prone to violence. This violence may in turn have contributed to their wives' passivity and their daughters' consent, and it may have influenced their need to conceal the incest. Herman and Hirsch (1981) also note that many of the victims in their sample felt abandoned by their mothers. The message that these mothers transmitted over and over to their daughters was "your father first, you second." The mother-daughter relations were often marked by frank and open hostility. In contrast, many daughters described their fathers in much more nurturant terms.

It is clear then that not only are incest families often characterized by volatile and stressful relationships, but these relationships may be perceived very differently by the various family members. For example, while fathers may present the relationship with their daughter in a positive light, daughters may in fact evaluate it very negatively.

To what extent can family therapy affect and improve these relationships, and to what extent does therapy affect all family members the same way? It is generally assumed that family therapy will improve family relations in incest families and lead to better communication skills (Giarretto, 1982). An earlier comparison of the parents in this study found that both mothers and fathers reported an improvement in perceived family relationships, although the actual family bonds had often been disrupted (Sagatun, 1982). But will family relationships improve for the daughter? A typical coping model for incest victims (as well as other victims) is to help victims change from an internal, self-blame model to an external, blame-the-perpetrator model (Janoff-Bulman & Frieze, 1983). However, in the father-daughter incest situation, the offender is the victim's own father. Learning to blame their fathers and/or mothers may assist victims in coping with their stress, but it may result in loss of parental support and a deterioration in the relationship between the daughter and the parents. Rather than improving the family relationships, at least as far as the daughters are concerned, the therapy may in fact serve to worsen the child-parent ties.

The consequences of incest may also be much more severe for the daughters than for the parents, and much harder for the victims to recover from. Sagatun (1984) found that victims of incest often suffer from posttraumatic stress symptoms long after the incestuous relationship has ended. Silver et al. (1983) argued that the betrayal of trust and the abuse of the parental role in incest relationships produce devastating effects on the social-psychological development of incest children. To what extent can therapy alter the perceived consequences of the incest for family members? Presumably, therapy should serve to lessen the traumatic impact for all members, but it may in fact have more positive effects on parents than on the victims.

Finally, this paper studies the effect of court-ordered therapy on the perceptions of family relationships and consequences before and after therapy. To what extent do the perceptions of family members under court order differ, and to what extent do their perceptions differ from the perceptions of those who are not ordered by a court to participate in therapy? One preliminary study found that offenders on court order were more likely than offenders who were voluntary participants to increase their reports of self-blame, and they tended to report more positive results from the therapy (Sagatun, 1981).

METHOD

Sample

Our sample consisted of 56 male incest offenders, 36 spouses, and 43 incest victims. All respondents were members of a Parents United program in a large urban area in California. Parents United is a self-help therapy group for incest families that operates in close conjunction with the county's child sexual abuse services. Of the offenders, 53 were fathers and 3 grandfathers. Similarly, 36 of the spouses were the mothers of the victims, and 3 were grandmothers. One of the daughters reported being a stepdaughter, 28.6% of the offenders reported being stepfathers, and 8.1% of the spouses reported being stepmothers. The mean age for fathers at the beginning of the incest was 39, while the mothers' mean age was 34. According to the fathers, the mean age for the daughters at the beginning of the relationship was 12.2, while the mothers reported the age to be 11 years, and daughters 11.5 years. Thirty-five percent of the fathers reported that they belonged to the middle class, 22.2% of the mothers reported a middle-class background, and 58.1% of the daughters described themselves as middle class. A relatively small percentage of the sample said that the father was unemployed at the time of the incest: 5.4% of the fathers, 2.8% of the mothers, and 14.0% of the daughters. The most frequent income category given by the fathers was in the $15,000-20,000 range, while both mothers and daughters indicated the $20,000-25,000 range most frequently. Among the fathers, 75% described themselves as white, 8.9% as Mexican American, and 5.4% as black and other groups. Among the mothers, 72.2% were white, 13.9% Mexican American, and

2.8% black and other groups. Among the daughters, 51.2% said that they were white, 16.3% Mexican American, and 11.6% black and other groups.

Questionnaire Instrument

A self-administered questionnaire was used to study the perceptions of family relationships and consequences before and after therapy. The respondents were asked to rate the family relationships on a 9-point scale where 1 was very good and 9 was very bad. To get the before-therapy measures the subjects were asked how they would describe the relationship at the "time of the incest." To get the after-therapy measures they were asked how they "now" would describe the relationship. In all they filled out six scales, all three relationships before and after therapy. They were also asked to rate the consequences of the incest before and after therapy on a similar scale. Finally, they were asked a series of background questions, including whether they were ordered by a court to participate in the therapy program.

Procedure

Permission was granted by the group leadership to ask members of the group to participate in the study. Participation was completely voluntary, and the members were assured that all their answers would be confidential. Both the therapy group and the Human Subjects Committee which approved the research proposal required that all subjects and the answers remain completely anonymous.

The self-administered questionnaire instrument was handed out to members during their therapy sessions. The sample consisted therefore of those members who were present during these sessions. Only one father refused to participate and did not allow his daughter and wife to respond.

As can be seen from the sample description, there were more offenders in the program than there were victims and mothers. Offenders were also more likely to be court ordered into therapy than other family members. Moreover, members of the same family did not necessarily participate in the same therapy sessions. This arrangement, combined with the fact that no family identifying information was allowed on the questionnaire, made it impossible to match the responses from members of the same family. The responses must therefore be seen as representing information on the three types of incest family members, rather than on individual members of the same family.

Design

This study included both a within- and between-groups design. The within-group comparison focused on the changes in perceptions of family relationships before and after therapy with each group. For example, the fathers' perceptions of the father-daughter relationship before therapy were compared with the fathers' perceptions of the father-daughter relationship after therapy. Similar comparisons were made for the other two groups. The between-groups comparison focused on the changes in family perceptions amongst the three groups before and after therapy. For example, a comparison was made of the fathers', mothers', and daughters' perceptions of the father-daughter relationship before therapy and after therapy.

In all, the perceptions of three different relationships — the father-daughter relationship, the mother-daughter relationship, and the mother-father relationship — were studied within and between groups before and after therapy. In addition, similar within- and between-group comparisons were made for the perceptions of the consequences of the incest on the family, both before and after therapy and for court-ordered and voluntary members.

RESULTS

Table 1 presents the between-groups comparisons of the perceptions of family relationships before and after therapy. Before therapy, only the father-daughter relationship was perceived in a significantly different way across the three groups. Fathers thought that the relationship was relatively good, mothers saw it as negative, and the daughters gave the relationship a poor rating. Fathers saw

Table 1

Between-Group Comparisons of Family Relations, Before and After Therapy

	Father $\overline{X}$	Mother $\overline{X}$	Daughter $\overline{X}$	F	df	p
			Before Therapy			
Father-daughter	3.5625	5.0833	6.5333	11.314	2	.0001*
(N)	(53)	(29)	(40)			
Mother-daughter	4.7667	4.0833	4.5938	.532	2	.589
(N)	(52)	(32)	(38)			
Mother-father	6.2252	4.5000	5.3571	.68	2	.508
(N)	(50)	(30)	(38)			
			After Therapy			
Father-daughter	3.344	4.167	6.2667	10.469	2	.0001*
(N)	(39)	(12)	(31)			
Mother-daughter	3.567	2.583	4.718	3.231	2	.045*
(N)	(30)	(12)	(33)			
Mother-father	4.032	2.667	5.357	4.356	2	.017*
(N)	(31)	(13)	(28)			

* significant finding

the mother-father relationship as the worst of the three, while both victims and mothers saw the father-daughter relationship as the worst in the family. It is important to note that while fathers saw the father-daughter relationship as the most positive in the family, the daughters gave it their worst rating.

After therapy, there were significant differences in the perceptions of all three relationships across the three response groups. The father-daughter relationship was reported as much better by the fathers than by mothers and daughters. The mothers reported the mother-daughter relationship as very good, the fathers saw it as somewhat positive, and the daughters saw it as neutral. The mother-father relationship after therapy was also perceived as good by the mothers, neutral by the fathers, and worse by the daughters. The daughters consistently perceived the family relationships after therapy as more negative than the parents. Again, the fathers gave their best rating to the father-daughter relationship, while the daughters gave it their worst rating.

Table 2 shows the within-group comparisons of the family relationships before and after therapy. We see that both the fathers' and mothers' ratings of the mother-daughter and the mother-father relationship improved significantly after therapy. None of the daughters' assessments of the family relationships improved.

Table 3 shows both the between and within comparisons of the perceived consequences of the incest for the family. We see that the family members differed significantly in their ratings of the consequences for the family after therapy, with the daughters giving the most negative ratings. All three groups perceived the consequences for the family as significantly worse before therapy than after therapy. However, the daughters still saw the consequences as quite negative even after therapy.

The effect of court order on the perceptions of family relationships are examined in Tables 4 and 5. There were no significant effects of court order on family perceptions before therapy. After therapy there were significant main effects both on the ratings of the father-daughter and the mother-daughter relationships, with mothers on court order particularly likely to rate the relationships as improved. There were no significant interaction effects.

The effects of court order on perceptions of consequences are listed in Table 6. Both fathers and mothers on court order were more likely to give negative ratings of the consequences at the time of the incest, but there were no significant interaction effects of family position and perceived consequences. There were no signifi-

Table 2

Within-Group Comparisons of Family Relations Before and After Therapy

	Before $\overline{x}$	After $\overline{x}$	t	df	p
		Father's Perceptions			
Father-daughter	3.5625	3.3438	6.42	31	.675
(N)	(32)				
Mother-daughter	4.7667	3.5667	2.25	29	.032*
(N)	(30)				
Mother-father	6.2252	4.0323	3.51	30	.001*
(N)	(31)				
		Mother's Perceptions			
Father-daughter	5.0833	4.1667	1.78	11	.102
(N)	(12)				
Mother-daughter	4.0833	2.5833	2.14	11	.056*
(N)	(12)				
Mother-father	4.5000	2.6667	2.28	11	.044*
(N)	(12)				
		Daughter's Perceptions			
Father-daughter	6.5333	6.2667	0.43	29	.669
(N)	(30)				
Mother-daughter	4.5938	4.7188	0.21	31	.837
(N)	(32)				
Mother-father	5.3571	5.3571	0.00	27	1.000
(N)	(28)				

* significant finding

Table 3

Between and Within Comparisons of Consequences Before and After Therapy

	Between					
	Father	Mother	Daughter	F	df	p
	$\overline{x}$	$\overline{x}$	$\overline{x}$			
Before therapy	7.355	7.250	7.118	0.078	2	.926
(N)	(31)	(12)	(34)			
After therapy	3.143	4.240	5.417	6.520	2	.002*
(N)	(41)	(25)	(36)			

	Within				
	Before	After	t	df	p
	$\overline{x}$	$\overline{x}$			
Father	7.3448	3.0345	7.65	28	.0001*
(N)	(29)				
Mother	7.8182	3.4545	6.44	10	.0001*
(N)	(11)				
Daughter	7.2121	5.3333	2.66	32	.012*
(N)	(33)				

*significant finding

Table 4

Effect of Court Order on Family Relations Before Therapy

	Court						Main Effects			Interaction Effects		
	Father		Mother		Daughter							
	Yes $\overline{X}$	No $\overline{X}$	Yes $\overline{X}$	No $\overline{X}$	Yes $\overline{X}$	No $\overline{X}$	F	df	p	F	df	p
Father-daughter	3.51	4.33	4.11	5.45	5.64	6.33	2.914	1	.091	.113	2	.894
(N)	(35)	(15)	(9)	(20)	(11)	(21)						
Mother-Daughter	5.00	4.80	4.00	4.50	3.90	4.65	.252	1	.617	.313	2	.732
(N)	(34)	(15)	(10)	(22)	(10)	(20)						
Mother-Father	6.44	5.80	5.67	5.52	5.40	5.75	.181	1	.671	.325	2	.724
(N)	(32)	(15)	(9)	(21)	(10)	(20)						

Table 5

Effect of Court Order on Family Relations After Therapy

	Court								Main Effects			Interaction Effects		
	Father		Mother		Daughter									
	Yes $\overline{x}$	No $\overline{x}$	Yes $\overline{x}$	No $\overline{x}$	Yes $\overline{x}$	No $\overline{x}$			F	df	p	F	df	p
Father-Daughter	3.17	3.50	1.50	4.70	3.67	7.31			11.488	1	.001*	2.731	2	.073
(N)	(24)	(6)	(2)	(10)	(9)	(16)								
Mother-Daughter	3.59	3.00	1.00	2.90	4.80	4.82			.004	1	.952	3.822	2	.542
(N)	(22)	(6)	(2)	(10)	(10)	(17)								
Mother-Father	3.87	4.33	1.67	2.80	2.50	6.47			7.174	1	.010*	2.238	2	.116
(N)	(23)	(6)	(3)	(8)	(8)	(15)								

* significant finding

Table 6

Effect of Court Order on Perceived Consequences

	Court						Main Effects			2-Interaction Effects		
	Father		Mother		Daughter							
	Yes $\bar{x}$	No $\bar{x}$	Yes $\bar{x}$	No $\bar{x}$	Yes $\bar{x}$	No $\bar{x}$	F	df	p	F	df	p
Before Therapy	7.70	6.83	8.50	7.00	6.55	7.29	.034	1	.854	.937	2	.397
(N)	(23)	(6)	(2)	(10)	(11)	(17)						
After Therapy	3.23	3.07	5.14	3.89	4.18	6.58	.399	1	.529	2.758	2	.068
(N)	(32)	(15)	(7)	(18)	(11)	(19)						

82

cant effects of court order on perceptions of consequences after therapy.

DISCUSSION

The results show that incest family members often perceive family relationships very differently. It appears that divergent perceptions of family relationships is a common factor in incest families. Such differential perceptions of their mutual relationships may further exacerbate the communication problems in incestuous families.

Before therapy, the father-daughter relationship received the most divergent ratings, with the offender and the victim differing the most in their perceptions. While the father saw the relationship as good, the daughters saw it as bad. Whether this relationship is rated as a "special one" (Spencer, 1978) or as a "hostile" relationship (Herman & Hirschman, 1977) may depend on *who* is giving the assessment. The divergent perceptions of the father-daughter relationship by the offender and the daughter may be an expression of ego-defensiveness. The father may try to "excuse" the sexual involvement by saying that the relationship was especially good. The daughters may feel that characterizing the relationship as especially "bad" puts the full blame on the father. Such ego-defensive tendencies, when accounting for a negative event, have been found to be quite prevalent, particularly in attribution research (Shaver, 1975). Sagatun and Prince (1984) found that even seemingly neutral background factors were described in an ego-defensive manner in incestuous families, in order to reflect more positively on the respondent.

While previous literature in the field has described the mother-daughter relationship as particularly estranged, this was not the case in these families. The mother-daughter relationship was seen as neutral by all family members at the time of the incest, and received the most similar ratings across family members. The father-mother relationship before therapy was given a particularly negative rating by fathers, perhaps reflecting a desire to "account" for the special relationship with the daughter.

After therapy, all three ratings of family relationships differed significantly across the three groups. This disparity is caused primarily by the daughters' failure to greatly improve their ratings after therapy. In contrast, both sets of parents significantly improved their ratings. Mothers, in particular, gave very good ratings to the relationships that they were directly involved in.

A major goal of therapy for incest victims is to improve the family relationships. The fact that therapy does not appear to have this effect on the victims is of great concern. Their low ratings may in fact reflect a basic dilemma in therapy for incest victims. This program, like many other therapy programs for victims (Fox & Scherl, 1972) encourages the victims to externalize the blame in order to diminish their own sense of guilt and shame. In many cases, this means blaming the offender rather than themselves. In the incest situation, the victims are told that they should not see themselves as the "seducers," but instead should hold the adults in the family responsible for the abuse. However, blaming the parents contributes to the continuation of stressful relations within the family; these relations may even worsen after therapy if this model is followed. While the offender may learn to assume personal responsibility in such therapy programs, he may also continue to feel resentment and anger toward the daughter for reporting the abuse and for blaming him for the relationship. Daughters blaming their mothers for not protecting them from their fathers may also generate a negative reaction. By helping victims to alleviate their own (misplaced) sense of guilt and wrongdoing, the therapy program may unwittingly make it even harder for the daughters to relate positively to their parents, particularly their fathers.

The clinical implication of this dilemma is that therapy programs somehow must find a way to diminish the victims' sense of self-blame and at the same time to improve the relationship between the victims and their parents. To recover from the incest trauma, the victims must gain the support of their significant others. Designers of therapy programs must therefore be aware of how the different models of reattributions for father, mother, and daughter interact, if they hope to produce a system that does not backfire. It is much easier to unilaterally blame an unknown rapist than an incest offender who is also one's father (Miller & Porter, 1983). A model that emphasizes placing blame on situational factors and transitory behaviors rather than on self or parents may prove to be the most beneficial for incest victims. Moreover, a therapy program that distinguishes between assigning blame for a past problem, and assuming responsibility for a future solution may also prove helpful (Brickman et al., 1982).

The issue of court-ordered therapy for incest families is hotly debated in many jurisdictions. In general, voluntary and self-directed therapy is thought to be more beneficial than forced therapy. Opponents of court-ordered therapy argue that a court order may encourage clients to "fake" an attitudinal change in order to please both counselors and the legal system. However, court-ordered therapy may be the only means to ensure that these families in fact receive appropriate treatment. Moreover, by forcing the members to participate, a court-ordered program may ensure that the participants stick with the treatment and reap the benefits of a continued program. The results reported here did not show many significant differences between court-ordered and non-court-ordered clients, especially in their perceptions after therapy. The social policy implication is that the authority of the court may safely be used to ensure treatment as a condition of probation and in addition to incarceration where appropriate.

The results of this study are weakened by small cell frequencies, a nonrandom sample, and the lack of an appropriate control group. Future research should attempt to alleviate all of these shortcomings. Although a large, random sample of incest families in therapy is hard to achieve, researchers should attempt to gather such a sample in order to ensure more reliable results. In addition to using a simple rating scale, other means of ascertaining the family relationships could also be included. To form a more complete picture of interpersonal perceptions and degree of accuracy in gauging other family members' feelings, research should also include reports on how family members think the other members perceive their interrelationships. Such patterns could then be compared to perceptions of family members in appropriate control groups.

Variations in the amount of time spent in therapy may confound the results, and the time period involved should be controlled for. Although we did have that information in this study, we did not use it as a control variable because of the already small cell frequencies. Similarly, a new study should attempt to record the perceptions of family relations at the onset of therapy, instead of relying on recollections.

Most important, future research needs to directly address the reasons for the relatively low improvement in the daughters' perceptions of family relations after therapy. By comparing the reactions to different therapeutic models involving different types of internal and external responsibility models, this research may be able to determine which types of therapy can best ensure an improvement both in the victims' self-esteem and family relationships. If at all possible, studying the reactions of intact family units would better aid this goal.

This study has shown that incest family members differ in their perceptions of family relationships, and that they differ significantly in their reactions to therapeutic intervention. It has demonstrated the importance of looking at the perceptions of each of the family members, in order to get a complete picture of the interpersonal dynamics in the incest family constellation. In has also implied that therapy programs must take into account the effects of individual coping models on family interactions, and that the reactions of significant others must be built into therapy strategies. Although individual coping models may have the desired effect on the clients' own self-esteem, interpersonal and environmental factors may counteract the positive gain. Hence, to achieve the double goal of improved individual self-esteem *and* improved family relationships, therapy models that are compatible for all family members need to be developed. The greater negative perceived consequences of incest among the daughters also indicate that particular care should be taken to alleviate the stress for the victims of incest.

REFERENCES

Anderson, L., & Shafer, G. (1979). The character-disordered family in community treatment model for sexual abuse. *American Journal of Orthopsychiatry, 49,* 436-445.

Brickman, P., Rabinowitz, V. C., Karuza, T., Coates, D., Cohn, E., & Kidder, L. (1982). Models of helping and coping. *American Psychologist, 37,* 368-384.

Browning, D. H., & Boatman, B. (1977). Incest: Children at risk. *American Journal of Psychiatry, 134,* 69-72.

Fox, S. S., & Scherl, D. J. (1982). Crisis intervention with victims of rape. *Social Work, 17,* 37-42.

Gentry, C. (1978). Incestuous abuse of children: The need for an objective overview. *Child Welfare, 57,* 354-364.

Giaretto, H. (1982). *Integrated treatment of child sexual abuse: A treatment and training manual.* Palo Alto, CA: Science and Behavior Books.

Herman, J., & Hirschman, L. (1977). Father-daughter incest. *Signs, 2,* 735-756.

Herman, J., & Hirschman, L. (1981). Families at risk for father-daughter incest. *American Journal of Psychiatry, 138,* 967-970.

Janoff-Bulman, R., & Frieze, I. H. (1983). A theoretical perspective for understanding reactions to victimization. *Journal of Social Issues, 39,* 1798-1809.

Kaufman, I., Peck, A., & Tagiuri, C. (1954). The family constellation and overt incestuous relations between father and daughter. *American Journal of Orthopsychiatry, 24,* 266-279.

Kock, M. (1980). Sexual abuse in children. *Adolescents, 15,* 643-648.

Lustig, N., Dresser, J. W., Spellman, S. W., & Murray, T. B. (1966). Incest: A family group survival pattern. *Archives of General Psychiatry, 14,* 31-40.

Miller, D. L., & Porter, C. A. (1983). Self-blame in victims of violence. *Journal of Social Issues, 39,* 139-153.

Raphling, D. L., Carpenter, B. L., & Davis, A. (1967). Incest: A genealogical study. *Archives of General Psychiatry, 16,* 505-511.

Sagatun, I. (1981). Court ordered therapy for incest offenders. *Journal of Offender Counseling, Services & Rehabilitation, 5,* 99-105.

Sagatun, I. (1982). Attributional effects of therapy with incestuous families. *Journal of Marriage and Family Therapy, 8,* 99-104.

Sagatun, I. (1984). Post-traumatic stress and coping in incest families. *Journal of Sociology and Social Welfare, 11,* 854-876.

Sagatun, I., & Prince, L. (1984). Incest families: Background and structure as perceived by different family members. Unpublished manuscript, Sociology Department, University of California, Riverside.

Shaver, K. (1975). *Introduction to attribution processes.* New York: Wintrop.

Silver, R., Boon, C., & Stones, M. (1983). Searching for meaning in misfortune: Making sense of incest. *Journal of Social Issues, 39,* 81-103.

Spencer, J. (1978). Father-daughter incest: A clinical view from the corrections field. *Child Welfare, 57*(9), 581-590.

Weiss, J., Rogers, E., Darwin, M. R., & Dutton, C. E. (1955). A study of girl sex victims. *Psychiatric Quarterly, 29,* 1-27.

Family Centered Casework Practice with Sexually Aggressive Children

John E. Henderson
Diana J. English
Ward R. MacKenzie

SUMMARY. A survey research project was conducted to collect data on 25 variables associated with sexually aggressive children and family centered casework practice in a public child welfare agency setting. The data was intended to provide a demographic description of the population and assess related casework practice methods in order to develop recommendations for change in agency policy and practice. The sample population was found to be a largely heterogeneous group. Demographic variables such as age at time of offense, history of victimization, criminal history, behaviors in placement, legal status, family composition, perpetrator/victim age differential confirm other research findings or present evidence for concern which was previously based on speculation. Casework practice methods were found to be inconsistent in identification, risk assessment, placement decisions, and case management. A casework model developed from practice experience literature review and oriented to family systems theory was presented in training to 158 casework staff. Post-training data collection was examined to determine possible effects of training. At post-training, casework staff demonstrated an improved ability to identify the sexually aggressive child.

Sexually aggressive youth and their families present the social worker with special challenges to casework practice and treatment methodology. This group of children includes the adolescent sexual offense perpetrator and the more recently acknowledged latency age child sexual offense perpetrator (Stickrod, 1987). A significant number of these perpetrators will not be adjudicated; these youth are without the benefit of intervention from the juvenile justice system, which some professionals view as at least integral to, if not required for, effective treatment and supervision (Dreiblatt, 1982). It is also widely held that when one is working with the sexually aggressive youth specialized skills and reliable assessment and decision-making methods are required to develop effective and appropriate case planning and treatment. Furthermore, there is growing evidence that successful intervention with sexually aggressive youth must address not only the individual's clinical treatment issues but also those found in the child's family and in legal and other related social systems (Becker & Abel, 1984; Groth & Loredo, 1981).

This study was developed in response to casework supervisors in a public child welfare agency identifying sexually aggressive children as presenting a major problem in day to day practice. A project committee of supervisors and caseworkers was organized to develop an issues paper, review current regional policy and practice, define sexually aggressive behavior, and examine placement resources and the related decision-making process. The committee would then propose recommendations for change in both agency policy and casework methodology.

In order to understand more fully the problems and needs of the sexually aggressive youth, the committee initiated a survey research project in a five county area. Data was collected on 25 variables associated with sexually aggressive children and family centered casework practice. The selection of cases to be studied and criteria for identifying appropriate cases is discussed in the Method section below. The results of this initial survey of cases in the five county area (N = 41) described a sample in many respects consistent with other demographic surveys of juvenile sexual offenders (Wasserman & Kappel, 1985). Some features, however, were seen as substantially associated with the agency context from which the sample was selected; for example, 70% of the children had been placed out of their family home. In general, the sample represented a heterogeneous group widely differentiated by virtue of age, family composition, offense typology, and other factors. Data analysis also found little consistency in casework methodology for assessing risk to reoffend, out-of-home placement decision making, and case planning. For example, some sexually aggressive children considered highly likely to re-offend were left in the home with their victims, and some children considered to have low likelihood of re-offending were placed in highly restrictive settings.

As a result of recommendations developed from analysis of the initial survey data, a staff training program was designed and presented to 158 agency staff. In addition to training, two part-time staff were designated to provide consultation on cases involving sexually aggressive youth. Data collection continued for the following six months on newly identified cases producing a post-training sample of 32. The pre/post groups were then compared in order to consider possible results of training and consultation and were consolidated to view the overall sample for demographic information.

The casework practice model presented in the staff training was influenced by a review of literature pertinent to the sexually aggressive child. The incidence and prevalence of adolescent sexual offenses has gained relatively substantial documentation (Ageton, 1983; Groth, 1977; Longo, 1982), although many believe the full extent of this problem has yet to be determined. Clinical work with the adult sexual offender often revealed a history of sexually aggressive behavior in evidence by twelve years of age. Similarly, clinical work with the adolescent is finding some youths who are able to ". . . identify, retrospectively, that their offending patterns of thinking and behavior began as early as age 5" (Ryan, G.). The training included a broad perspective of possible age ranges, from six to seventeen years, within which sexually aggressive behaviors were believed to be potentially possible.

One important limitation found in reviewing the literature is that treatment models almost exclusively address adjudicated youth and assume that probation services and court supervision are available. This brought into question the applicability or suitability of some of these treatment methods in a noncriminal court system setting.

Many of the treatment programs which serve the adolescent perpetrator share similar components or clinical focus such as assisting the youth in acknowledging and taking responsibility for the offense, restructuring cognitive distortions, training in social skills, utilizing group processes to address denial and minimization, providing sex education and victim treatment, and working with the family system (Knopp, 1985). The emphasis on family systems theory as this relates to both etiology and remediation of sexually aggressive behaviors is receiving increasing recognition (Boniello, 1986; Lankester & Meyer, 1986; Monastersky, 1982; Sgroi, 1982). Behaviorally oriented treatment components are often essential for those youth who have established a deviant arousal pattern; and techniques may include covert desensitization, masturbatory satiation, and aversive conditioning. These techniques have in large part been adapted from work with adult sexual offenders (Abel et al., 1984).

While caseworkers in the public agency will usually not be providing direct clinical services, they must be familiar with and be able to arrange appropriate treatment from qualified providers. The caseworker will need to have the skill and ability to identify the sexually aggressive child. The caseworker's role must include the capacity to act in an assertive and directive role in circumstances wherein often the child's and family's pathology may characterize itself through denial, minimization, and retreat from intervention. The caseworker's intervention in the family system will often have a direct impact on the potential for remediation and must reflect treatment, supervision, and victim protection priorities.

This project is designed to improve casework practice methodology in a public child welfare agency providing services to sexually aggressive youth and their families. Dependent variables targeted for change are foster care placement rates and decision making for foster care placement. Criterion measures will consider cases differentiated by the perpetrator's level of risk to re-offend and whether a potential victim does or does not reside in the home. Post-training utilization of a risk assessment device and decision tree is expected to reduce placement rates for some types of cases. A more consistent relationship between level of risk to re-offend, the presence or absence of potential victims in the home, and a decision to place or not to place out of home should be evident in the post-training group as compared to the pre-training group. It is also anticipated that staff training in identification and assessment of sexually aggressive youth will result in more frequent identification of cases and in a larger portion of identified youth being in younger age groups. Finally, training and consultation are expected to improve the type and rate of services caseworkers arrange for the sexually aggressive youth in terms of services directly related to treatment needs. There is also an expectation that other variables included in data collection may reflect change as an indirect result of training or may be the result of a larger sample demonstrating a more normal distribution of characteristics. For example, if average age decreases, it might be anticipated that nonadjudicated youth will represent a larger portion within the sample.

METHOD

This study utilized a research survey design to gather data on the incidence, distribution, and relationship between certain variables. These variables included subject variables related to identified sexually aggressive youth as well as those variables associated with casework practice, client services, adjudication, and victim characteristics. The purpose of the study was to describe and document both the target population and related casework practice methods in order to develop sound policy and practice recommendations towards the sexually aggressive youth.

The initial data analysis of 41 cases identified a substantial need for staff training and education. Project staff proposed training program in conjunction with specialized case consultation as a means to better address the needs of the client population and to work towards resolution of some of the problems identified with casework methodology. These proposals were supported by agency management and the project went forward with the development and implementation of both training and consultation services. Post-training data collection resumed and created an opportunity for a time-ordered criterion from which to consider change in the pre-/post-training data.

Subjects

The survey population was defined as any child from six through seventeen years who had received any services from the agency during the last year and who was exhibiting sexually aggressive behavior, either at the time of referral or when this behavior became evident while the case was in an active ongoing status. Behavioral descriptors for sexually aggressive behaviors were adopted from definitions developed by Caren Monastersky, formerly with the University of Washington Juvenile Sex Offender Project, and Lucy Berliner from the Harborview Hospital Sexual Assault Center in Seattle, Washington. Criteria described sexual contact as touching of genitals and/or intercourse with aggression being defined as physical force used to accomplish the act. Coercive sexual contact accomplished by direct or implied threat of harm to gain compliance or prevent report was included in the construct definition of aggression. Coercion could also be implied through inequality in physical size, age differential, developmental sophistication, or deception if used to gain compliance or prevent reporting. To some extent, these criteria are present in Washington criminal statute; however, legal definitions of sex crimes might additionally require findings of culpability and sexual gratification. For purposes of this study, neither culpability nor adjudication were required criteria and the sample broadly included criminal offenders and nonadjudicated sexually aggressive children from ages six to seventeen.

Forty-one pre-training cases were identified from the five county area which included rural, suburban, and urban populations. During the six month post-training period, 32 new intake cases were identified by caseworkers or their supervisors.

Material

The instrument used for data collection was a 25 item questionnaire prepared by two project staff and reviewed by the project committee. A risk assessment scale including perpetrator, victim, and family characteristics was developed and utilized for assessing level of risk to re-offend.

Procedure

The Project Director contacted each Casework Supervisor in the region, explained the purpose and parameters of the study, enlisted their support, and developed a list of identified cases. Data collection was completed by project staff's reading case files and interviewing assigned caseworkers. The case count was limited to cases that had been active within the last year. Fifty-three pre-training cases were identified by caseworkers or their supervisors. Eight cases were eliminated after review as the child's behavior or circumstances did not meet the established definition for sexually aggressive behavior.

Survey data was reviewed, and recommendations for change in casework practice and policy were proposed. These recommendations included a staff training program directed towards case management issues believed to have been illuminated by the data analysis. Data, as well as impressions gathered from interviews with caseworkers, suggested a need for education and orientation to differentiated typologies of sexually aggressive behaviors. Recognizing differences in case characteristics would enable the caseworker to develop prescriptive intervention plans responsive to the particular needs of the child. There appeared to be inconsistent practice in out-of-home placement decision making in relation to assessed risk to re-offend and in potential victims residing in the same homes as the perpetrators. Often an absence of case planning by qualified therapists to ensure treatment for the sexually aggressive behaviors was found.

Project staff and committee members developed a one-day training program which was presented to a total of 158 caseworkers, supervisors, and managers in small groups of fifteen to twenty-five participants. The training was mandatory and included virtually all casework service staff and their supervisors. The content of training provided an overview of pertinent literature including normative and deviant sexuality, values clarification related to sexuality, and sexually aggressive behaviors from both personal and professional perspectives, case management and treatment within the context of family systems theory, including behavioral, cognitive, and social skills, and sex education components.

Training also introduced the use of practice tools including a Risk Assessment Protocol consisting of a checklist with perpetrator, family, and victim risk criteria each to be rated on a five-point Likert-type scale. Categories for risk related variables were adopted in part from the "Juvenile Sexual Offender Decision Criteria" checklist developed by staff of the Juvenile Sexual Offender Program at the University of Washington Hospital, Adolescent Clinic, in Seattle (Wenet & Clark, 1977). An out-of-home placement planning form and process was used to train towards appropriate and consistent decision making, and a case planning matrix which identified differentiated levels of intervention based on the assessed level of risk to re-offend in intrafamily sexual abuse cases was also used. The need to utilize specialized and qualified providers for diagnostic and treatment services was also addressed. Finally, the training concluded with group exercises utilizing the new model with prepared case examples.

In addition to the training, two part-time consultants were assigned to the region, and they began providing case consultation services to caseworkers as new intake cases were identified. The consultants assisted with the risk assessment and case planning process as well as with collection of post-training data. The formal project ended approximately six months post-training, at which time the post-training sample was at 32 cases.

RESULTS

A total sample of 73 cases was included in the study with data on 25 variables collected for each case. Forty-two cases were identified prior to training and 31 post-training. As this study was originally designed for survey purposes, the resulting data does not lend itself to an analysis by inferential statistics. Nonetheless, some results are reported in terms of pre/post frequencies and percentages. Changes in pre/post samples cannot be examined for statistically sound correlations to training and consultation, however, it is reasonable to observe these changes as moving toward an improved state of casework practice and representing a more thorough and appropriate inclusion of children previously under-reported and under-served.

Age of Child at Time of Reported Offense

The majority (80%) of perpetrators identified in the pre-training group were in the adolescent age range. Post-training data illustrates a substantial and significant shift towards representing a larger portion (34.3%) of children under the age of twelve (see Table I).

Table I

Age of Child at Time of Sexually Aggressive Behavior

	Pre-Training		Post-Training		Combined	
Age by Years	N	%	N	%	N	%
6-8	2	4.9	3	9.3	5	6.8
9-12	6	14.6	8	25.0	14	19.2
13-14	24	58.5	11	34.4	35	47.9
16-17	9	21.9	10	31.3	19	26.1
Totals	41	100	32	100	73	100

While the majority of perpetrators remain in the adolescent age range, the preadolescent age group may continue to under-reported despite its larger representation in the post-training group. Research and treatment with adolescent perpetrators are beginning to uncover childhood histories which suggest that sexually aggressive behaviors are often in evidence at eight or ten years of age. Just as work with adult sexual offenders helped point out the prevalence of adolescent sexual offenses, work with the adolescent sexual offender often appears to point to earlier sexual aggressive behavior. This information may provide a clearer view of etiological sources, and it speaks strongly towards efforts aimed at early identification and intervention.

Perpetrator's History of Sexual Victimization

Data on the history of victimization was reported during caseworker interviews or in case file records often noted as information provided by the parent(s). Post-training data identified 75% of the children as having been sexually victimized; whereas pre-training data found 56.1% with victim histories as seen in Table II. The risk

Table II

Perpetrator History of Being Sexually Abused

	Pre-Training		Post-Training		Combined	
	N	%	N	%	N	%
Perpetrator had history	23	56.1	24	75	47	64.4
Perpetrator did not have history	17	41.5	4	12.5	21	28.8
Missing Value, unknown	1	2.4	4	12.5	5	6.8
Totals	41	100	32	100	73	100

assessment device utilized in training included victim history as one factor to be considered in predicting risk to re-offend. Training and utilization of the risk assessment tool appear to have resulted in increased awareness and documentation of victim history. The increase in reported victimization may also be related to a younger age group post-training.

Family Composition

Although changes in data from pre- to post-training were evident in virtually every category, it is difficult to interpret the findings with respect to training. The combined sample were represented by biological parents in 15.1% of the families; single parents were 31.5%; blended (with stepparent), 28.8%; adoptive parents, 9.6%; and foster care placements, 12.3%. It is important to acknowledge these different family compositions in light of a growing emphasis on family system theories which identify the family as a "stage" from which the child acts out in a sexually aggressive way (Boniello, 1986). The dynamics associated with different family systems are seen to be related to planning for effective case management and treatment interventions.

Case examples used in the staff training pointed out how services could directly address treatment issues for the family and for the sexually aggressive youth. For example, a circumstance commonly found in sibling incest was an older sibling baby-sitting for a younger sibling with the older child assuming a parental role in the single parent family. The older child's offending behaviors in this situation are interpreted by some clinicians as an expression of resentment for being required to fulfill a parent's role and as a method to eventually create conflict between the mother and older child in order to create distance in their inappropriate relationship (Lankester & Meyer, 1985). If this family has day-care services made available to it, the victim can be protected, while the older sibling is enabled to assume a more appropriate role within the family and to have more time to develop age-appropriate social contacts. The mother arranges care for one child without relying on the other child to fill a caretaker role.

Perpetrator to Victim Age Differential

Findings in this area remained relatively consistent across the pre- to post-training groups. The fact that 58.6% of the victims were more than five years younger than the perpetrator, while 36.6% were less than five years younger is not of interest. This reflects a group of younger perpetrators whose victims' ages tend to be in closer proximity to their own ages. Quite often literature that focuses on adolescent sexual offenders remarks that the age differential between the perpetrator and victim is one of several appropriate criteria useful in distinguishing normal experimental curiosity from deviant or abnormal sexually aggressive behavior (Deisher et al., 1982; Groth, 1977; Groth & Loredo, 1980). However, if we consider the younger children who are exhibiting sexually aggressive behaviors, their victims are likely to be closer to the same age as the perpetrator. Due to closer age proximity between the preadolescent perpetrators and the victims, age differential may sometimes be a less significant assessment issue. Stickrod (cited in Ryan, 1987) has drafted a definition and descriptive criteria for the "young child perpetrator" which does not rely on age differential to distinguish sexually aggressive behavior.

Out-of-Home Placement

The pre-training sample group experienced 73.1% out-of-home placements compared to a 59.4% placement rate in the post-training group. Two office areas within the region which prior to training had practiced a more categorical policy of placing sexually aggressive children experienced in excess of a 30% reduction in placement rates.

Further analysis of the placement rates was considered in terms of correlations between placement rates, level of risk to re-offend and the presence or absence of potential victims in the perpetrator's home. There was a noticeable reduction of placements in circumstances which included an assessed low risk to re-offend and a potential victim present in the perpetrator's home. The casework model presented in training provided guidelines to placement including the presence of a functioning adult ally in the home, the degree of victim trauma, the availability and utilization of services such as day care and treatment by the family, and the extent to which the perpetrator acknowledged his or her offense and cooperated with treatment and supervision requirements. For cases which met this criteria, the perpetrator was often able to return to or remain in the home.

Another area of change, as noted in Figure I, was evident in those cases where risk to re-offend was moderate but where there was not a potential victim in the home. In the post-training sample, no such identified cases resulted in out-of-home placement. While placement rates for high risk offenders who had potential victims in their home remained the highest in the overall population, a consistent percentage, 10% of the total group, continued to live at home with a potential victim.

Placement decisions were principally associated with conflicts or risks related to sexually aggressive behavior; however, this was not

Placement by Risk and Potential In-home Victim

Figure I. Placement by risk to re-offend and potential victim in the home or absence of potential victim in the home.

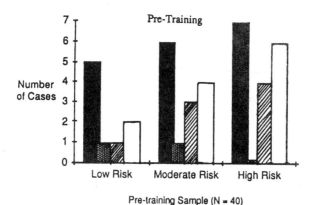

Pre-training Sample (N = 40)

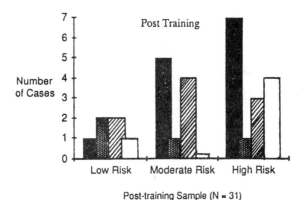

Post-training Sample (N = 31)

NOTE

- ■ Placement, victim (potential) in home
- ▨ No placement, victim (potential) in home
- ▦ No placement, no victim (potential) in home
- ☐ Placement, no victim (potential) in home

always the case. For example, a low risk perpetrator with no potential victim in the home may have been placed due to severe family conflict or due to his or her own abuse experienced in the home. In those cases where a seemingly inappropriate combination of factors was present, the placement status may not reflect a decision by the caseworker but may reflect instead circumstances of the case. A juvenile offender may have completed a court-ordered period of community supervision before his or her treatment needs have been met with the family's "support" decline to continue in treatment. Unless the youth's parents request a placement or they can be found neglectful of protecting the potential victim in the home, placement may not be an option.

Legal Status

The legal status of the sexually aggressive youth beyond the context of criminal court is particularly relevant to the child welfare agency and case management decisions and responsibilities. Approximately 29% of the pre-training group were nonadjudicated, while in the post-training group 62.5% were nonadjudicated. This reflects the first group's average age which represented older youth who were more frequently adjudicated. The post-training group was represented with a larger portion of perpetrators under the age of twelve who generally are not adjudicated. In Washington State, criminal prosecution of children under twelve years of age must first establish culpability; and except in unusual and chronic cases, this is generally not a common practice. Other situations involving older youth may find substantiated sexually aggressive behavior; however, by the nature or circumstances, the case cannot or will not be prosecuted. This takes on particular significance if one accepts the general thesis of the treatment community that the optimum method to keep offenders in treatment, or to induce a suppression effect, is to prosecute and hold the individual accountable. If this is true, then a sizeable number of sexually aggressive children in the community are without these constraints. There is discussion in the literature (Drieblatt, 1982), supported by observations of caseworkers, that some form of structure and supervision is often indicated for the sexually aggressive youth and family. Some degree of authority may be required in order to overcome denial and resistance to intervention. While the implied or actual authority of the public agency may be adequate in many cases to facilitate treatment and intervention compliance, the agency is presented with sexually aggressive children who are a high risk to others including siblings and who themselves and/or their families are resistant to intervention. In the absence of criminal sanctions and court influence, the required structure and authority to ensure treatment and supervision may be the responsibility of the public agency worker to pursue through the family courts. The issue of parents being considered "neglectful" in terms of not seeking treatment for a nonadjudicated sexually aggressive child as this might create potential risk to a sibling is a complicated matter that will need to be addressed by the courts.

Other findings of particular significance compared criminal charges to actual behavior. In approximately 54% of all the cases which were charged, the eventual conviction by the court was for a less serious offense than was indicated by the described behavior. Typically, acts of penetration (rape of varying degree) were convicted at levels of indecent liberties, that is, sexual contact without penetration.

Criminal Histories and Behaviors in Placement

Data in these areas may address some of the misconceptions associated with sexually aggressive youth, while suggesting a certain typology of more predictably serious and chronic offenders. Between 60% and 80% respectively of the pre- and post-groups had no criminal history. Similarly, a large percentage of both groups, up to 60%, were reported as not having significant behavior problems in the home or in out-of-home placement. Significant behavior problems were described by category and were identified primarily in terms of when those behaviors precipitated failure in foster or family placement.

About half of those youth who had victim related criminal histories prior to the identified sexual acting out were reported to continue to exhibit assaultive and/or sexually aggressive behaviors afterwards. When cases were grouped by those including a high risk assessment, prior- and post-assaultive or sexually aggressive behaviors and criminal histories, and problems in placement, only about 10% of the total samples fit this profile. It became evident during interviews with caseworkers that these more severely disturbed youth had chronic histories of placement disruption, and treatment efforts became virtually impossible due to the child's instability. In this comparatively small group of sexually aggressive youth, community based and nonrestrictive foster care placements cannot be expected to meet the youths' treatment needs or provide protection of potential victims in the community.

Victim/Perpetrator Relationship

In the overall sample, approximately half of the victims and perpetrators were family members living in the same home. In the group sample prior to training, a large percentage, 26.8%, of the victims were known to the perpetrator but did not live in the same home. The pre-training group was characterized as somewhat older with longer case histories. The post-training sample group was somewhat younger than the first with shorter or recently initiated case histories. This post-training group reported a much lower percentage of offending outside of the home; the victims were generally in closer proximity to the perpetrator by relationship and shared living circumstances. Generally speaking, only ten percent approximately, of the group, offended against unknown victims. This argues for a comprehensive assessment of the risks presented within the family by the presence of a child identified as sexually aggressive; other siblings may be potential victims, if not already victims, of prior sexual aggressions.

Perpetrator's Number of Victims

In the overall sample, 43% of the perpetrators were reported to have had one victim; 50% were reported to have had between two to five victims. It has been found that the adult sexual offender may commit in excess of 300 sex crimes during his lifetime (Abel et al., 1984). There is a growing body of evidence that the offender's history of multiple offenses and multiple victims has started at twelve years of age or before (Awad, Saunders & Levene, 1979; Longo, 1982). Multiple victims implies that behavioral patterns are being reinforced and that even with the young perpetrators treatment may have to address well-established deviant behaviors and cognitive distortions which have enabled the child to become sexually aggressive. Early intervention with sexually aggressive youth has primarily been directed towards the adolescent child with the hope of reducing a potential development of chronic deviant behavior. It may be a painful discovery to find that the adolescent child may already have a history of multiple victims and that "early intervention" for this youth should have come much sooner.

DISCUSSION

The survey research portion of this project was largely successful in describing the sexually aggressive youth as they are represented in a sample from one region in a state child welfare agency. Data collection results in general support previous findings in terms of the perpetrator's own history of victimization, age at first reported offense, victim/perpetrator relationship, and other similar demographic features. The study adds documentation to mounting recognition and concern for pre-adolescent children who are victimizing other children. These younger perpetrators are currently identified in circumstances found true for the adolescent some ten or fifteen years ago. That is, their problem is just gaining recognition; treatment expertise is rare; and treatment resources are almost nonexistent. Many social workers involved with young children and their families will themselves need to seek specialized training which addresses assessment and treatment methods relevant to the pre-adolescent sexually aggressive child. Moreover, the social work profession should take a proactive role in encouraging recognition of the incidence of sexually aggressive behaviors among pre-adolescent children. If some of these young children are in the early stages of developing a chronic and deviant problem which might eventually impact over 300 victims, early intervention is clearly a necessary priority.

A comparatively small group of perpetrators, mostly older adolescents have committed the bulk of sexual and nonsexual criminal offenses reported for this sample and have chronic histories of multiple foster care placements. In the early 1970s, Washington State juvenile criminal codes were changed in part to protect "incorrigible" or "status offender" children from being place in secure settings with juvenile criminal offenders. The result observed by many has been an increase in runaways and "street kids," some of whom are sexually aggressive youth with current or prior histories of adjudicated offenses. In simple terms, these youth will not and cannot be served in a least-restrictive, nonsecure setting as is now required by state law. Both the state and federal lawmakers must reassess the impact of both the Youth Services Act and parallel state legislation, which has created a population of street children beyond the supervisory reach of the adult community.

The results of training and consultation appear to have benefited both identification and placement processes. For those children in placement, more offense-specific treatment services were arranged for the primary clients and their families. This may have been influenced considerably by the process of the project committee and consultants, who identified resources and the consultant's role in assisting with risk assessments and placement decisions.

It is important to acknowledge the considerable disparity in case practice methods observed for the pre-training as well as post-training groups, although this disparity was less evident in the post-training group. Caseworkers described widely differing perspectives in terms of their views of children's psycho/sexual development, normative and deviant sexual behaviors, and assessed trauma to the victim. Others expressed considerable discomfort in working with sexually aggressive children or expressed a preference to work with nonoffending youth. The casework supervisor should acknowledge that some social workers bring childhood experiences of their own which may influence their perception of either the victim, perpetrator, or parents. While training may be expected to produce general improvement in casework practice, such as identification of sexually aggressive children, the casework supervisor will need to match the special skills and interest of particular caseworkers to the exceptional case management and treatment needs of the sexually aggressive youth. Designating specialized staff in each local office or work unit to consult with other caseworkers or to be assigned those cases identified as involving sexually aggressive youth would be helpful.

In conclusion, these findings emphasize the need for additional recognition of and work with preadolescent children. Further research on the etiology of sexually aggressive behaviors may benefit from a perspective including early childhood development. Intervention with the preadolescent child, who is not usually served by the juvenile courts, will require new strategies from the professional community, family courts, and public child welfare agencies.

REFERENCES

Abel, G. G., Becker, J. V., Cunningham-Rather, J., Rouleau, J. L., Kaplan, M., & Reich, J. (1984). *Treatment of child molesters* (available from Columbia University, SBC-TM, 722 West 168th St., Box 17, New York, NY 10032).

Ageton, S. (1983). *Sexual assault among adolescents.* Lexington, MA: Lexington Books.

Awad, G. A., Saunders, E., & Levene, J. (1979). A clinical study of male adolescent sex offenders. *International Journal of Offender Therapy and Comparative Criminology, 28* (2), 105-116.

Becker, J. V. & Abel, G. G. (1984). *Methodological and ethical issues in evaluating and treating adolescent sexual offenders* (NIMH Monograph, June 1984).

Boniello, M. J. (1986). *Connections Magazine*, pp. 4, 5, 20.

Deisher, R. W., Wenet, G. A., Paperny, D. M., Clark, T. S., & Fehrenbach, P. A. (1982). Adolescent sexual offense behavior: The role of the physician. *Journal of Adolescent Health Care, 2*, 279-286.

Drieblatt, I. S. (May 1982). *Issues in the evaluation of the sex offender.* Paper presented at the Washington State Psychological Association Meetings.

Broth, A. N. (1977). The adolescent sexual offender and his prey. *International Journal of Offender Therapy and Comparative Criminology, 21*, 249-254.

Groth, A. N. (1977). The adolescent sexual offender and his prey. *International Journal of Offender Therapy and Comparative Criminology, 21*, 249-254.

Groth, A. N. & Loredo, C. M. (1980). Juvenile sexual offenders: Guidelines for assessment. *International Journal of Offender Therapy and Comparative Criminology, 25*, 31-39.

Knopp, F. H. (January 1985). *Remedial intervention in adolescent sex offenses: Nine program descriptions* (available from Safer Society Press, 3049 East Genesee St., Syracuse, NY 13224).

Lankester, M. A. & Meyer, W. (1986). *Relationship of family structure to sex offense behavior.* Unpublished manuscript.

Longo, R. E. (1982). Sexual learning and experience among adolescent sexual

Child Protective Service Workers' Ratings of Likely Emotional Trauma to Child Sexual Abuse Victims

Diana J. English
Linda G. Tosti-Lane

SUMMARY. One hundred fifty-four child welfare workers were asked to rate the likely emotional trauma to victims of child sexual abuse. Each caseworker rated twelve scenarios in which the child victim was sexually assaulted by another child. Ratings were made on a scale of 1 (low risk of emotional trauma) to 10 (high risk of emotional trauma). The research literature suggests that these caseworkers' assessments of the example cases were uniformly incorrect. One out of every three caseworkers either over- or underrated the likelihood of emotional trauma in no less than eight of the scenarios. One in five of the caseworkers over or under rated all twelve of the scenarios. The inconsistencies revealed in this preliminary study suggest that a more refined study of caseworkers' assessment of trauma is needed. Also training must be developed for caseworkers and community professionals who assess emotional trauma in the course of developing treatment and caseplans.

INTRODUCTION

Quality and consistency of casework service in public agencies are major practice issues of the 1980s. Each protective service client ought to receive a consistent comprehensive assessment, is entitled to protection and should be referred to appropriate levels of service based on need. Services to the family should also minimize further victimization to the child. This study examines the consistency of casework practice in a child welfare agency related to a segment of the child sexual abuse population. Specifically, this study relates to children who are sexually abused by other children.

Questions regarding the consistency of caseworker assessment of likely emotional trauma to child sexual abuse victims developed in the context of a larger research study focusing on caseworker evaluations of child perpetrators' likelihood of reoffending. In the perpetrator study we developed an assessment of risk tool that included a victim vulnerability scale. One item in the victim vulnerability scale related to the degree of trauma experienced by the child. Caseworker evaluation of likely emotional trauma to victims in the perpetrator study was so inconsistent that we were unable to use the data to draw any valid conclusions. Estimation of likely trauma to victims is a critical part of perpetrator assessment. Accurate information related to the harm experienced by the victim and the acts of the perpetrator is critical to casework decisions related to services to the victim, removal of the perpetrator and to family reunification. The inconsistency discovered in the earlier study caused some concern among project staff.

An accurate estimate of likely emotional trauma to the child victim is related to several decision making points in case assessment and service delivery. The level of emotional and physical harm the victim has suffered is related to service delivery during crisis intervention, when making decisions regarding protection, and when making decisions regarding perpetrator contact and family reunification. Lastly, there is the question of referral of service after the initial disclosure crisis has been resolved. Information regarding anticipated short- and long-term effects of physical and emotional abuse must be related to the caretaker who will have ongoing contact with the child. When possible, a plan to ameliorate effects of abuse should be developed and carried out.

REVIEW OF THE LITERATURE

Prevalence

The actual incidence and prevalence of child sexual abuse, in the family and outside of the family, are unknown. National studies indicate an estimated rate of 0.7 cases of child sexual exploitation per 1,000 children per year (National Center on Child Abuse and Neglect, 1981). This rate includes children who have been sexually abused by adults and by other children both within and outside the child's home environment.

Despite little concrete information on prevalence, reports of child sexual abuse have steadily increased over the last decade (Russell, 1983). In 1981 between 10-15% of cases referred to child protective services in Washington state were cases with allegations of child sexual abuse. In 1986 at least 11,000 referrals, approximately 25% percent of all child protective services, were cases alleging child sexual abuse. Whether the actual incidence of sexual abuse is on the rise, or whether the increase is due to better community understanding of the problem and therefore more referrals, is unknown. We do know from early work such as that done by Kinsey, that many women in the 1950s reported sexual abuse in their early childhood years.

Nearly 15% of all child sexual abuse referrals are identified as third party sexual abuse (Washington State Department of Social and Health Services, 1981-1986). Third party cases are those situations where the alleged perpetrator of an abusive act does not live in the same home as the child, and there is a functioning adult ally available to protect the child. For third party cases the agency provides an information and referral service to families and reports the abuse to law enforcement agencies for further action. The remaining 85% of child sexual abuse cases are primarily intrafamilial child sexual abuse. These cases included situations where there are adult perpetrators and child victims, and situations where there are child perpetrators and child victims. Services in these cases involve assessment of protection issues and referral to appropriate services.

An unknown proportion of the cases alleging sexual abuse referred to child protective services each year are sexual abuse cases where the perpetrator is also a child. A child perpetrator is defined as any male or female under the age of eighteen who has committed an illegal sexual act against another child. While the actual proportion of adult perpetrator to child perpetrator is unknown, recent research indicates that as many as 50% of child sexual abuse victims seen in sexual assault clinics in Washington have been sexually assaulted by other children (Deisher, Wenet, Paperny, Clark, & Fehrenbach, 1982). A recent study in Washington state indicated that 73 child perpetrators had more than 150 child victims within a one-year period (English, Henderson, & McKenzie, in press).

Physical vs. Emotional Trauma

Research also indicates that child sexual abuse victims may experience differential physical and emotional trauma in connection with the experience of sexual abuse. Caseworkers and parents make initial decisions about whether to seek physical treatment for victims of sexual abuse. These decisions are based on type of abuse, whether there are any physical signs of injury, verbal reports of injury or hurt by victims, and/or law enforcement need to collect evidence. Referral issues related to emotional trauma experienced as a result of the sexual abuse are more difficult to assess.

The literature indicates that there may or may not be obvious behavioral signs of emotional trauma related to the abuse. It is theorized that emotional effects of sexual abuse are related to elements of sexualization, betrayal, feelings of powerlessness and loss of self-esteem (Adams-Tucker, 1982; Finkelhor & Browne, 1985). Another potential source of emotional trauma to child victims is the reaction of those with whom the child comes into contact once the sexual abuse has been disclosed. Children who are not believed, who are unprotected, ridiculed or blamed are more likely to experience emotional trauma than child victims who are believed, protected and supported (Finkelhor & Browne, 1985; Gomes-Schwartz, Horowitz, & Sauzier, 1985). The presence of an adult functioning ally is critical to the reduction of emotional abuse to a child who has been the victim of sexual abuse (Lewis & Sarrell, 1969; Sgroi, 1982). The child's developmental age also can be a predictor of the emotional trauma in that the very young child is less able to understand the sexual nature of the abuse and therefore the child may experience less emotional trauma (Gelinas, 1983; Gomes-Schwartz et al., 1985). Lastly, the child's reaction to the abusive situation can be exacerbated by a service system which over- and underreacts to the situation (Berliner & Stevens, 1986; Finkelhor & Browne, 1985).

In recent years much attention has been focused on service to victims which emphasizes believing the child and ensuring support and protection (Berliner & Stevens, 1986; Sgroi, 1982). Casework practice has to some extent incorporated these ideals, and more sensitive approaches to child sexual abuse cases have been developed by caseworkers, law enforcement personnel and prosecutors. These efforts should be supported. However, less attention has been paid to the likely emotional trauma to victims, and how this type of assessment might affect case decision-making. The current assumption is that all children experience a high degree of trauma if they have been sexually abused. Recent research indicates that child sexual abuse victims experience a range of reactions to the abuse that can include obvious signs of distress to severe emotional distress indicated by behavioral acting out (Brooks, 1985). Research also indicates that effects of abuse may be different for different developmental stages. Emotional trauma in particular needs to be assessed in relation to other factors present before and after the sexual abuse itself (Finkelhor & Browne, 1985; Mrazek & Mrazek, 1981).

Typically, caseworkers see their major role as one of referring the child victim to therapeutic specialists for assessment and treatment. While referral of a child sexual abuse victim to therapeutic specialists for assessment is an appropriate case outcome, the reality is that caseworkers must frequently make case decisions before a professional evaluation has been completed. In fact, in many instances, caseworkers may be the only other professional involved in the case. Given that caseworkers are involved in the situation at crisis, as well as through crisis resolution, there is an important opportunity to reduce the likelihood of further trauma to victims by supporting functioning adult allies and by making accurate initial assessments of the immediate service needs of the child based on level of likely emotional trauma present at the time of intake.

The purpose of this study was to develop some preliminary evaluation of the consistency of caseworker ratings of likely emotional trauma to children who had been sexually abused by other children.

METHODOLOGY

Construction of Case Examples

Twelve cases representing typical child perpetrator/child sexual abuse victim situations routinely referred to the agency were developed. A panel of child protective service caseworkers from a five-county area, who routinely provide services to child sexual abuse cases, were requested to submit typical child perpetrator/child victim sexual abuse cases currently on their caseload. Case examples included situations where older adolescents sexually assaulted younger victims, same-age children engaged in sexual acts together, males aggressed females, males aggressed males, and females aggressed males.

The literature on child sexual abuse was reviewed and derived ratings were developed for each of 12 case examples. Two of the caseworkers on the project had specialized expertise and training in the area of child sexual abuse and victimization. These two caseworkers reviewed each case example and developed a derived rating for each case example based on experience and information available from the literature review. The derived ratings were specified as a possible range with 1 being low likelihood of emotional trauma and 10 being a high likelihood of emotional trauma. Criterion used in the assignment of ratings included child's age, level of trauma such as use of force, level of intrusiveness, frequency of abuse, relationship of perpetrator to victim, and the reaction of primary caretaker. The project staff then compared the range scores they individually derived and, where differences occurred, agreement was reached for the final tool.

The use of a range of scores for each example, rather than one score, was utilized because the project staff felt that the circumstances in any given case situation could vary depending on individual case characteristics to such an extent that flexibility in choosing the level of likely emotional trauma was necessary. However, given differences that reflect the need for a range, it was also felt that there should also be limits to the likely range based on the actual circumstances being evaluated. For example, in case number 10, the information provided does not clearly state whether penetration actually occurred, or whether the parent/caretaker believed the victim. If penetration had not occurred and if there was a functioning adult ally, the case may have been rated at the lower end of the range. If, however, penetration had occurred, and/or if the parent did not believe the victim, rating of likely emotional trauma to the victim would have been toward the higher end of the range.

Table 1 shows the data collection instrument used in the study.

TABLE 1

Data Collection Instrument

For the following exercise, you are to assess how traumatic the sexual abuse/exploitational situation is to the child on a scale of "1" to "10" being the highest. You are not assessing risk, but the emotional trauma to the child that the situation presents.

_____ 1. A five-year-old boy was fondled three to four times by his 19-year-old live-in uncle. Mother believes child.

_____ 2. A three and a half-year-old female has sexual intercourse with 14-year-old developmentally disabled child. She is having recurring nightmares.

_____ 3. A 15-year-old developmentally disabled girl is raped one time by her father's cousin. Father denies abuse occurred. Mother doesn't know who to believe. Her 17-year-old cousin threatened to hurt her dog.

_____ 4. A five-year-old female is touched by her 15-year-old babysitter. Mother believes and doesn't allow babysitter back over.

_____ 5. An eight-year-old girl's 17-year-old brother repeatedly shows the child pornographic pictures of other children.

_____ 6. A 12-year-old boy reports that his friend's 17-year-old sister played the "I dare you game" and had him put his penis in her vagina.

_____ 7. A one-year-old boy is fondled and has anal intercourse attempted two to three times by his babysitter.

_____ 8. An eight-year-old boy is stopped in the woods near his play house. His 13-year-old neighbor forces him to pull his pants down and sucks his penis.

_____ 9. Three preschoolers (ages 3, 3 1/2, and 4) are asked to play doctor by their 10-year-old playmate. He puts sticks up their vaginas causing minor tears on the vaginal walls. The mothers believe their daughters.

_____ 10. A 13-year-old girl reported to her mother that the neighbor's 18-year-old brother was playing with her and her friend. Part of the game she and her friend were playing with the brother was that he got to put his penis in their vaginas because they were playing "chicken."

_____11. A four-year-old reports that her 12-year-old brother walks into her room when the parents are gone and he opens his bathrobe with nothing on underneath. He tells her not to tell mom and dad. This happened a number of times.

_____12. Two eight-year-old children are observed by a neighbor looking out the window. They are engaging in simulated sex with their clothes on.

Generally, derived ratings at the lower end of the range were given to case examples where there was a combination of factors such as no evident injury, fondling or exposure as opposed to penetration, a one time occurrence perpetrated by an individual outside the family structure, and whether the child had a functioning adult ally who was available to provide support. Higher ratings were given to case examples where the reverse was true, that is, that there was a combination of factors that could include injury, penetration, multiple occurrences of the abuse, assault by a family member, and no functioning adult ally present to provide support to the child. See Table 2 for trauma factors included in each case example. Individual factors present in each example contributing to the likely emotional trauma to the victim varied from example to example. In some cases, information on a particular factor was not present, resulting in a wider range in the derived score.

Since this study was exploratory in nature and used in the context of caseworker training, no specific hypotheses were developed. It was expected, however, based on data from the perpetrator study, that caseworker ratings would be inconsistent. The question was whether the level of inconsistency was sufficient to warrant additional, more rigorous research.

Subject Selection and Administration of Case Examples

The 12 case examples were administered to 154 child welfare caseworkers who practice in one of six regions in Washington state. All caseworkers in a five-county/seven-office geographical area who provide protective service and reconciliation services to fam-

Table 2

Trauma Factors Included in Case Development

Derived Rating	Use of Force		Level of Intrusiveness		Frequency		Relationship to Perpet.		Reaction of Primary	
	Pain/inj.	No inj.	Pene-tration	Non-Pene-tration	1 time	1 or more times	family of member	outside of family	Believe	No Info./don't
#1 (3-6)		X		X		X	X		X	
#2 (5-9)	X		X		X			X	?	
#3 (8-10)	X		X		X		X			X
#4 (2-5)		X		X	X			X	X	
#5 (3-5)		X		X		X	X			?
#6 (3-8)		X	X		X			X		?
#7 (2-6)		X		X		X		X		?
#8 (4-8)		X		X	X			X		
#9 (4-8)	X		X		X			X	X	
#10 (3-8)		X	X	?	X			X		?
#11 (2-5)		X		X		X	X			
#12 (1-2)		X		X	X			X		?

X = factor included in the case example

? = unclear whether factor is present or not

117

ilies with perpetrators and victims in the home were included in the study.

During eight training sessions, agency caseworkers were asked to rate the likely level of emotional harm experienced by the victim in each case example. Ratings were to be made on a scale of 1 to 10 with 1 being very low likelihood of emotional trauma, 5 being a moderate likelihood of emotional trauma, and 10 being very high likelihood of emotional trauma. After rating the case examples, each caseworker was given the derived ratings based on the literature review for each case example as well as the range and median score for each case example within their own training group. Differences between derived scores and scores within each group were used as a basis for discussion and consensus building concerning likely emotional trauma to victims.

In small group exercises, caseworkers were asked to identify the reasons they assessed a particular level of likely emotional trauma to the victim in each example, and why their ratings might differ from the modal ratings or individual ratings within their own groups. A summary of the literature supporting each of the derived ratings was presented to the large group as part of individual group ratings as compared to within- and between-group ratings.

DATA ANALYSIS

One hundred and forty-seven responses for each case example were collected and analyzed. The design of the study and the composition of each training group did not allow for complex data analysis. The data were primarily analyzed based on frequency and percents of the total group responses for each case example. See Table 3 for a chart indicating within-range, above-range and below-range scores for each case example. The results of the ratings were uniformly inconsistent. One in five caseworkers rated all 12 of the case examples outside the range of likely emotional trauma to the victim in each scenario as supported by the literature. In 8 of 12 case examples, one in three caseworkers rated the likely emotional trauma to the victim outside the derived range. Ratings outside the derived range were both under- and overrated, with a varying range of ratings outside the range for different case examples. However, the

Table 3

Caseworker Ratings of Likely Emotional Trauma to Victims by Case Example

| | | | Caseworker's Ratings | | | | | | |
| Derived Range | Within Range | | Below Range | | Above Range | | Total Out of Range | |
	N	%	N	%	N	%	N	%
#1 (3-6)	93	66	18	12	32	22	50	34
#2 (5-9)	80	64	0	0	67	46	67	46
#3 (8-10)	125	85	19	13	0	0	19	13
#4 (2-5)	107	73	16	11	18	12	34	23
#5 (3-5)	64	44	17	12	61	41	78	53
#6 (3-8)	120	82	8	5	19	13	27	18
#7 (2-6)	67	46	2	1	78	53	80	54
#8 (4-8)	88	60	1	1	57	29	56	40
#9 (4-8)	98	67	8	5	41	28	49	33
#10 (3-8)	115	78	5	3	27	18	32	21
#11 (2-5)	97	66	2	1	48	33	50	34
#12 (1-2)	76	52	0	0	71	48	71	48

most frequent response (in the majority of cases) was to overrate likelihood of emotional trauma to victims.

Caseworkers were most consistent in identifying likely emotional trauma to victims in those case situations where there was clear evidence of forceful sexual abuse such as rape, and in cases where victims engaged in "I dare you" games. The least consistent ratings on case examples were at opposite ends of the spectrum. In one case, 53% of the workers overrated the likely emotional harm to the victim in a scenario where two eight-year-old children are fully clothed and engaged in simulated sex. Twenty-five percent of the respondents rated the likely level of emotional trauma at the moderate level, while 16% rated at the very high level. The second scenario that received the highest overrated score was a situation where a one-year-old child is fondled by an adolescent baby sitter. The perpetrator also "attempted intercourse." In this scenario the caseworker could be focusing on the attempted intercourse and the feeling of powerlessness the infant could have by being "covered" by a larger body. Physically, the infant could be having pleasurable sensations associated with manual manipulation related to the fondling. It must be remembered, though, that the caseworkers were asked to rate emotional trauma not physical trauma. The child could have residual emotional reaction due to pain, but this age child does not have the developed cognitive ability to associate abuse with the main contributors to emotional trauma, that is, sexualization, betrayal or stigma (Finkelhor & Browne, 1985; Gomes-Schwartz, Horowitz, & Sauzier, 1985).

DISCUSSION

The original findings of inconsistency in caseworker ratings of likely emotional trauma to child victims who are sexually abused by child perpetrators were reconfirmed in this exploratory study. Despite the shortcomings of the research design, the variance in ratings for the case examples was consistently out of range, and large enough to support the idea that caseworkers, at least in this situation, are inconsistent in assessing risk levels of emotional trauma to victims. Inconsistent assessment of emotional trauma is likely to result in different levels of service, and differential reactions to the abuse. Inconsistency may result in some children who need immediate services not being referred at the appropriate time and some children who may not need immediate interventions being referred too quickly. In either event, children may be further victimized by the service delivery system designed to assist and protect them.

Another implication related to the underlying differential response to child victims is that information, as well as referral, may be inappropriate and inadequate. Advising a parent that a child is likely to be severely traumatized by a situation, which may only result in moderate trauma and then only at a later developmental or minimal stage, could stimulate a parent to overreact. Parental overreaction may inadvertently stigmatize the child. On the other hand, underrating likely emotional trauma, resulting in inadequate information given to primary caretakers, may result in a child not receiving service intervention in a timely manner.

Some victim advocates criticize caseworkers for failing to validate a child victim's experience and thus further stigmatizing the child. However, we also know that children are traumatized by separation from their families as well as by loss of support by adult allies. Additionally, caseworkers by law, and by policy, are required to undertake reasonable efforts prior to separation of child and family. Caseworkers must balance these concerns and develop plans in "the best interest of the child." The actual incident of sexual abuse is only one of several factors contributing to emotional trauma. Caseworkers must consider all three factors in assessment and decision-making.

The inconsistencies found in this study may reflect some genuine differences of opinion among casework staff concerning likely emotional trauma to the victim based on field experience. For example, ongoing child welfare workers may rate likely emotional trauma to victims higher because they see the long term effects of abuse. On the other hand, caseworkers may rate likely trauma high based on their own personal experiences and/or attitudes toward sexually aggressive behaviors. Whatever the reason for the inconsistency in assessment in the initial disclosure of cases, research indicates that emotional trauma may resurface for resolution at different developmental stages and should therefore be expected and planned for in each case plan.

Another explanation for the inconsistency may be related to the method by which the case examples were developed. A more systematic approach to developing examples would have increased the value of the study. Nevertheless the case examples were designed to represent current types of cases received by child welfare caseworkers. The case examples were, in fact, derived from open cases, and should be representative of scenarios in which caseworkers frequently make critical decisions concerning perpetrators and victims. Even if additional review increased or lowered the derived ratings, the inconsistency would still be present in the assessment of likely emotional trauma to the child in the majority of examples. The results of this study indicate a level of inconsistency in current practice of assessment related to child perpetrator/child victim sexual abuse cases. Further study is needed. A posttest in this study would have helped answer the question of whether the agency training resulted in actual change in casework practice related to assessment of likely emotional trauma.

Current practice models in adult perpetrator/child victim sexual abuse cases are quite sophisticated, although they focus primarily on father/daughter incest cases. In recent years, increased attention to this area of practice has resulted in protocols and guidelines that give clear direction, specific practice procedures and decision guidelines regarding removal of a child victim from the home, conditions for visitation and treatment needs. Much less attention has been directed toward response systems directly related to issues of child perpetrator/child victim sexual abuse cases. In adult perpetrator/child victim cases the legal system is involved, meaning greater controls, resources and supports available. This is not the case in child perpetrator/child victim cases.

The Washington perpetrator study revealed that 45% of the child perpetrators were not adjudicated (English et al., in press). The main reason child perpetrators were not adjudicated was because the victim was unable to testify or the perpetrator was under the age of 12. In either case, similar behavior in adults or an older child most frequently results in adjudication, incarceration and referral for treatment. Even if a child perpetrator is adjudicated, they were most frequently undercharged. In other words, the charge for which they were convicted did not reflect the actual behaviors exhibited in the offense situation.

Inappropriate adjudication or lack of adjudication means that service providers, whether through the courts or child protective services, have less formal controls over the child. Most frequently this means that unless a family and/or the child perpetrator voluntarily agree to treatment, and pay for it themselves, little formal intervention will occur in these cases. Caseworkers in public child welfare agencies are frequently the first professionals involved in the discovery and disclosure of child perpetrator/child victim sexual abuse cases. Caseworkers in public child welfare agencies may frequently be the only professionals involved in service delivery to these families, whether perpetrator families or victim families. Given the critical involvement of caseworkers in these cases, it would seem appropriate that our training and policies reflect the best practice procedures.

If the discussion in the literature is valid, that is, the effects of sexual abuse are differential and frequently delayed, then the training of supervisors and caseworkers and the development of guidelines and standards for investigation should be developed. Such training should include refined assessment skills for both physical and emotional effects of sexual abuse, and a better understanding of the dynamics of emotional trauma. Caseworkers must have information on appropriate, as opposed to inappropriate and deviant, sexual behaviors in children and the relationship that emotional trauma has at different developmental stages. Lastly, an understanding of service needs for children experiencing the effects of child perpetrator/child victim sexual abuse should be more clearly articulated. Treatment referrals should be geared to specific problems present in the child victim and the child perpetrator, with the goal of restoring either child to normal functioning as well as alleviating differential victimization.

These preliminary findings indicate a need for a more refined study of caseworkers' assessment of likely trauma to victims. Attention should also be paid to service delivery issues once the assessment has been completed. Exploration of the most efficient and appropriate assessment and service delivery practices for these special situations should occur and guidelines developed. Lastly, training must be developed for caseworkers and other community professionals who are engaged in the process of assessing emotional trauma to victims.

REFERENCES

Adams-Tucker, C. (1982). Proximate effects of sexual abuse in childhood: A report on 28 children. *American Journal of Psychiatry, 139*(10), 1252-1256.

Berliner, L., & Stevens, D. (1986). Clinical issues in child sexual abuse. *Journal of Social Work & Human Sexuality, 5*, 93-107.

Brooks, B. (1985). Sexually abused children and adolescent identity development. *American Journal of Psychotherapy, 23*(3), 407-409.

Deisher, R. W., Wenet, G. A., Paperny, D. M., Clark, T. S., & Fehrenbach, P. A. (1982). Adolescent sexual offense behavior: The role of the physician. *Journal of Adolescent Health Care, 2*, 279-286.

English, D. J., Henderson, J., & McKenzie, W. (in press). Sexually aggressive youth: A study of service need. *Journal of Social Work & Human Sexuality.*

Finkelhor, D., & Browne, A. (1985). The traumatic impact of child sexual abuse: A conceptualization. *American Journal of Orthopsychiatry, 55*(4), 530-541.

Gelinas, D. J. (1983). The persisting negative effects of incest. *Psychiatry, 46*, 312-332.

Gomes-Schwartz, B., Horowitz, J. M., & Sauzier, M. (1985). Severity of emotional distress among sexually abused preschool, school-age, and adolescent children. *Hospital and Community Psychiatry, 36*(5), 503-508.

Lewis, M., & Sarrell, P. M. (1969). Some psychological aspects of seduction, incest and rape. *Journal of the American Academy of Child Psychiatry, 8*, 606-619.

Mrazek, P. B., & Mrazek, D. A. (1981). The effects of child sexual abuse: Methodological considerations. In P. B. Mrazek and C. H. Kempe (Eds.), *Sexually abused children and their families* (pp. 235-245). New York: Pergamon Press.

National Center on Child Abuse and Neglect (1981). *National study of the incidence and severity of child abuse and severity of child abuse and neglect* (DHHS Publication No. 81-30325). Washington, DC: U.S. Government Printing Office.

Russell, D. E. H. (1983). The incidence and prevalence of intrafamilial and extrafamilial sexual abuse of female children. *Child Abuse and Neglect, 7*, 133-146.

Sgroi, S. M. (1982). An approach to case management. *Handbook of Clinical Intervention in Child Sexual Abuse* (pp. 81-108). Lexington, MA: Lexington Books.

Washington State Department of Social and Health Services (1981-1986). (Monthly management report #122 a and b, and #124 a and b.) Unpublished raw data.

Relapse Prevention:
A Cognitive-Behavioral Model
for Treatment of the Rapist
and Child Molester

Craig Nelson
Michael Miner
Janice Marques
Kabe Russell
John Achterkirchen

SUMMARY. The treatment of sexual aggressives (i.e., rapists and child molesters) is aimed not at "curing" the offender but at helping the individual to control his behavior. The concept of control involves the active participation of the offender in a behavior change process and reinforces the fact that continued abstinence from offending requires the offender's continued attention. This paper describes Relapse Prevention (RP), a cognitive-behavioral model for helping the sex offender to gain control over his behavior, thus preventing the occurrence of a reoffense. RP attempts to help the offender maintain abstinence by identifying the decisions that place him at risk for offending (apparently irrelevant decisions, or AIDs), the situations that threaten his sense of self-control over his sexual behavior (high-risk situations), and the cognitive and affective precipitants in his offense pattern. Through multimodal techniques, this perspective proposes to assist offenders in enhancing control of their behavior by improving strategies to cope with their offense pattern. Specific RP assessment and treatment procedures are presented with an accompanying case illustration of their application.

The authors wish to thank Diana Fox, Joseph Murphy, and Marci Parlet for their help in the preparation of this manuscript.

125

It is, of course, the goal of any treatment program for sex offenders, regardless of its emphasis or orientation, to assist the offender in not reoffending. Individualized and specific goals such as modifying deviant sexual arousal patterns, remediating social and sexual skills deficits, improving affect management, heightening empathy toward others, enhancing self-esteem, promoting increased impulse control, and a host of other relevant objectives serve only as subgoals oriented toward aiding the offender in the ultimate task of abstaining from illicit sexual acts in the future. In her descriptive study of adult sex offender treatment programs, Knopp (1984) characterized specialists in the field as eschewing the term "cure" in favor of that of "control" of the deviant sexual behavior. The notion of cure implies that the problem has been resolved and no longer exists. Therefore, it means that the offender is neither at risk to relapse into previous offending habits nor in need of specific methods for avoiding a reoffense. Control, on the other hand, denotes that the problem is being restrained and curbed. It implies that the offender must take an active and vigilant role in managing a pattern of nonoffense. It is not unusual for an offender to believe earnestly that he will never molest or rape again, only to be caught by surprise when he finds himself in a tempting predicament that elicits a return of his deviant urges.

Because the treatment goal for all sex offenders is the maintenance of control over the prohibited sexual behavior, approaches for enhancing this maintenance must be implemented. As in sexually aggressive behavior, the problem of relapse or the full return to a former habit has also been identified as a major difficulty in the treatment of a variety of addictive behaviors (Brownell, Marlatt, Lichtenstein, & Wilson, 1986; Marlatt, 1985a; Marlatt & Gordon, 1980). One approach that has been developed in the field of addictive behaviors to deal with this problem is Relapse Prevention (RP) (Marlatt, 1985a; Marlatt & Gordon, 1980). RP is a self-control training program designed to help people maintain behavioral changes by anticipating and coping with the problem of relapse. The RP model has been previously adapted and proposed as a means to increase the maintenance of control of sexually aggressive behavior (Marques, Pithers, & Marlatt, 1984; Pithers, Marques, Gibat, & Marlatt, 1983). It is the purpose of this paper to further describe how this treatment approach can be implemented with rapists and child molesters both to initiate behavior change and to encourage its continued maintenance.

ASSUMPTIONS UNDERLYING APPLICATION OF RELAPSE PREVENTION

The analogy between sexual offending and other addictive behaviors is not novel, and the similarity has been previously noted by others (Knopp, 1984). Carnes (1983, 1984), for instance, has formulated a treatment approach for what he terms "sexual addicts." Unlike this approach, however, the application of the RP model does not assume that sexual offending is necessarily "addicting." The model is based on the premise that important similarities exist between certain sex offenders and other individuals with "indulgent" behavior problems (e.g., abuse of alcohol and other drugs, smoking, overeating, and compulsive gambling). This category of problem behaviors is defined as those acts which (a) lead to a state of immediate gratification; and (b) are followed by delayed negative consequences. Clearly, these characteristics are present in the indulgent behavior of sexual offending. A rape or child molestation leads to immediate gratification in the form of feelings of power and control over the victim, release of tension, and/or sexual gratification. These immediate positive feelings are followed by delayed negative consequences such as social disapproval, shame, guilt, and/or incarceration.

An important assumption in the application and extension of the RP model to the treatment of sexual aggressives is that there are common behavioral, affective, and cognitive components associated with the relapse process itself. One is an unpleasant emotional state that immediately precedes losing control and re-engaging in the indulgent behavior. Another is that the offender thinks about or plans to engage in the forbidden behavior before the indulgent behavior itself reoccurs. The Queen's Bench Foundation (1976) reported that nearly 77% of rapists in their study reported feeling frustrated, depressed, angry, or rejected before their attacks. Over two-thirds of the rapists in this study reported thinking about rape before committing their sexual attacks. Several sex offenders interviewed at Atascadero State Hospital reported a common sequence of events which led up to their offenses. First, the offenders found themselves in stressful situations with which they were unable to cope effectively. As a result, they began to feel negative emotions, such as anger, frustration, or anxiety. They then began to fantasize about performing the deviant sexual act. The fantasies evolved into thoughts or actual plans in the next step of the sequence. Finally, thoughts were manifested in the commission of the offenses. A similar pattern of thoughts, feelings, and behaviors leading to reoffense in sexual aggressives has been reported by others (Pithers et al., 1983). This sequence of stressful situation — no coping response — negative affect — fantasy — thought/plan — behavior fits closely the pattern reported by alcoholics, smokers, and heroin addicts who have relapsed (Marlatt & Gordon, 1980). Fantasy, however, appeared to play a more central role in the relapse process for sex offenders than has been reported for substance abusers (Marques et al., 1984).

COGNITIVE-BEHAVIORAL MODEL OF RELAPSE

Whether an offender will maintain control over his sexual behavior is, according to this model, determined by factors embedded in the relapse process illustrated in Figure 1. After the initial behavior change, an offender has a sense of self-efficacy and control over the behavior, as well as an expectation that he will continue to succeed in his goal of abstinence. This is the point at which many offenders are able to state to themselves and others that they are convinced they will not reoffend. According to the theory, this state continues until the offenders encounter a high-risk situation, that is any situation that threatens their sense of control over the indulgent behavior and increases the risk of reoffense. Although risk factors are individual for each offender, the authors have detected, in clinical work with both rapists and child molesters, several common elements: for example, the presence of a potential victim, the use of disinhibitors such as alcohol and drugs, negative affective states such as anger or frustration, interpersonal conflict, and rationalizations or justifications for engaging in the illicit sexual behavior. The degree of threat

FIGURE 1

COGNITIVE-BEHAVIORAL MODEL OF REOFFENSE

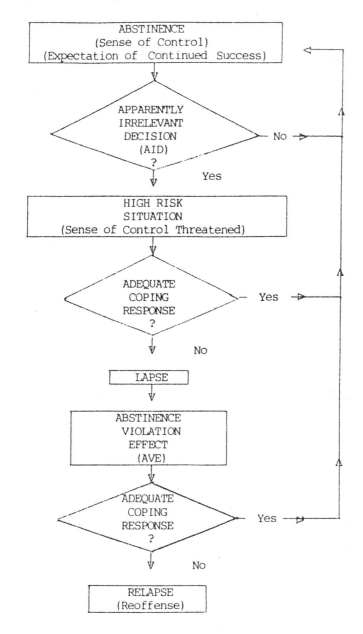

posed by any high-risk situation is related to the number, strength, and combination of the factors present.

An offender may proceed from the point of abstinence, with its associated sense of control and expectation of continued success, in a variety of ways. Some offenders have had difficulty avoiding or anticipating the high-risk situations in which relapse eventually occurred. Frequently, however, offenders appear to set the stage for their offense or reoffense by covertly seeking out high-risk situations (Marques et al., 1984; Pithers et al., 1983). For example, the abstinent pedophile who volunteers to teach a Sunday school class at his local church or the rapist who stops to pick up a female hitchhiker have both precipitated a potential high-risk situation. Such actions are labeled as "apparently irrelevant decisions" (AIDs)[1] (Marlatt, 1985c; Marlatt & Gordon, 1980). Through denial and rationalization, the offender places himself in extremely tempting situations which allow him to justify his crime by being overwhelmed and unable to resist the high-risk elements of the circumstances. Two major characteristics appear to identify an AID. First, the action appears rational, reasonable, or even worthy of praise. It is difficult to fault one, for example, for teaching Sunday school or aiding a hitchhiker. Secondly, the action places the individual in a high-risk situation that threatens his continued abstinence. Therefore, the decision merely appears irrelevant; in fact, it is quite relevant in the process of setting the stage for reoffense.

Once the offender encounters a high-risk situation, whether unavoidable or surreptitiously arranged through an AID, the ability to make an immediate coping response decreases the potential for the situation to provoke a relapse. Conversely, if a coping response is not made or is unsuccessful, the high-risk situation continues to carry the risk for offense. Thus, the danger or risk in any situation is inversely related to the degree to which one adequately copes with the predicament. At its simplest level, an adequate coping response may consist of avoidance or escape, that is, evading potential circumstances that would threaten one's sense of control or immediately withdrawing when such a situation is encountered.

A successful coping response will, by definition, reduce the chances of relapse and reoffense. In addition, the individual's self-efficacy, his expectancy for continued success (Bandura, 1977), is enhanced. If, on the other hand, no effective coping response is produced, the individual lapses in his abstinence. The notion of a lapse implies a slip or mistake that can be corrected, not that control is completely lost and the former undesirable behavior (sexual aggression) reoccurs. In the RP approach, a lapse is contrasted with a relapse in which control is completely lost and the previous pattern of undesirable behavior resumes. A lapse is seen as an important process or step that can, but does not have to, lead to total relapse. In the field of addictions, the lapse is the first instance of the forbidden or undesirable behavior. It may be the first cigarette for the abstaining smoker, the first drink for the abstaining drinker, or consuming too many calories for the dieter. As relapse is defined, in the case of sexual aggression, as the commission of an illicit sexual act, the lapse becomes whatever immediately precedes the offense. Concretely, the lapse may be the fantasy of the illicit sexual act (Pithers et al., 1983), experiencing sexual arousal in response to a deviant theme or object, actively seeking a potential victim, or the initial phases of the seduction of a child. The lapse is viewed as an individualized event, depending on the typical pattern and mode of operation of each offender. It is a cognitive, affective, or behavioral "danger signal" or "red flag" that a full-blown relapse is approaching. The response to the lapse determines whether the individual will return to abstinence or proceed to a relapse (Brownell et al., 1986; Marlatt, 1985c; Marlatt & Gordon, 1980).

Whether a lapse ultimately precipitates a return to the sexual offense depends upon a factor that has been labeled the "abstinence violation effect" (AVE). It consists of the cognitive and affective reactions to the occurrence of an initial slip or lapse following a period of abstinence. The AVE represents the conflict between the offender's previous self-image as an abstainer and his recent experience of the prohibited thought or action: "If I am no longer a sex offender, why am I masturbating to fantasies of children?" or "Why am I cruising, looking for women to rape?" As a result of the AVE, the offender experiences cognitive dissonance (Festinger, 1957) over the disparity between his beliefs about himself as an abstainer and the occurrence of a behavior that is directly incongruent with this self-image. Engaging in the prohibited behavior is one way to decrease the experienced dissonance. Another possibility is to reduce the dissonance by cognitively altering the self-image to bring it in line with the new behavior ("I guess I will always be a sex offender and there's no use fighting it"). Either strategy increases the probability that the lapse will escalate into a full relapse.

A second component of the AVE is a self-attribution effect. Rather than looking at the lapse as a unique response to a particularly difficult situation, the offender is likely to blame the act on his own deficiencies, (e.g., lack of willpower, internal weakness, a failure in his treatment). If the lapse is construed as a personal failure, the offender's expectancy for continued failure will increase (Abramson, Seligman, & Teasdale, 1978), thereby decreasing the resistance to subsequent lapses. The overall result is an increased probability that a lapse will be followed by a complete relapse (Marlatt, 1985a; Marlatt & Gordon, 1980; Marques et al., 1984; Pithers et al., 1983). The AVE is a dimensional phenomenon, not an all-or-none reaction. The greater the AVE, the greater the probability of relapse. If, on the other hand, the offender is prepared for a potential lapse, the AVE can be diminished and the offender can institute appropriate coping responses that may return him to continued abstinence.

A case of a 36-year-old child molester with whom the authors are familiar illustrates the relapse process. The offender began a pattern of molesting younger girls when he was a teenager. Shortly after his marriage in his early 20s, he was arrested for molestation and incarcerated in a residential treatment facility where he received a combination of intensive marital counseling and assertiveness training. After two years of this treatment, he was released upon the recommendation of the treatment staff. In reviewing his earlier treatment experience, the offender indicated that at the time of his release he viewed himself as "cured" and no longer at risk for reoffense. Although unclear about the rationale behind his previous treatment, the offender believed that as long as he listened to his wife and followed her direction he would have no more desire to molest. For approximately five years, he viewed his life as running smoothly and reported no return of his previous urges for molesting (abstinence). As his marital relationship began to deteriorate (stress) in the sixth year after his discharge, he began to spend increasing amounts of time in community activities that involved his daughter and other children (AID). He noted particularly enjoying the attention and esteem the youngsters directed at him. On several occasions, he started supervising the children when no other adults were present (high-risk situation). On one such occasion, he began horse-playing very physically with one of the girls in a swimming pool. Consequently, he became sexually aroused and interpreted the child's actions as seductive toward him (lapse). In response to this arousal, he reported feeling ashamed, depressed, and powerless (AVE) to prevent himself from molesting the victim (relapse).

The RP model assumes that the sex offender can learn to recognize the sequence or chain of events that precede a relapse, and can evolve appropriate coping strategies to intervene before it is too late. Offenders come to recognize that their offenses are neither isolated nor discrete events. Rather, they are the culmination of a long series of events, some of which are external (e.g., access to a victim, interpersonal conflict, substance abuse) and some of which are internal (i.e., affective states and cognitions).

RELAPSE PREVENTION ASSESSMENT PROCESS

From an RP perspective, treatment and assessment are closely wedded. The identification of factors contributing to the overall offense pattern, such as high-risk situations or deficits in specific coping abilities, are in themselves viewed as interventions of significance. Therefore, the dichotomy presented in this description between treatment and assessment is, to an extent, an artificial one made for purposes of explanation. The RP model does not view sex offenses as simple or isolated events. Rather, rape and child molestation are seen as complex behaviors with multiple determinants ranging from broad characterological factors to more circumscribed skill deficits and deviant sexual arousal patterns. Encompassing this broad range of determinants requires the comprehensive evaluation of a host of factors.

The main technique for highlighting this offense sequence or pattern is the development of individualized, detailed cognitive-behavioral offense chains. In the authors' experience, this is best accomplished by starting at the offense and moving backward in time, identifying each significant incident preceding the crime. This is first done for external events, and then the cognitive interpretations and affective responses to those events are added. This process helps the offender to separate his reactions to the events from the events themselves. In this way the cognitive distortions and irrational cognitions (e.g., "The child was being seductive towards me" or "Any woman who dresses that way in public is asking to have sex") become apparent. Each step, or link, in the chain is evaluated for its significance and relevance by having the offender determine whether it moved him closer to or away from committing the rape or molestation. This process, though tedious, produces a step-by-step sequence that clearly evolves into the offense. In other words, it becomes clear to both the therapist and the offender how these elements combined to result in the sexual aggression.

The process of constructing a cognitive-behavioral chain places the offender in the role of "making sense" out of his offense. If, however, the cognitive-behavioral chains do not clearly lead to the aggressive act, this suggests that there have been major omissions in the chain.

In addition to exploring offenses that have already been committed, the offender is asked to create an imaginary situation that could provoke a relapse/reoffense in the future; that is, he constructs a guided relapse fantasy (Marques et al., 1984; Pithers et al., 1983). Supplemental chains can be framed around the scenes elicited in guided relapse fantasies. From the chains of both actual and fantasized offenses, AIDs, high-risk situations, coping response failures, lapses, and AVEs are identified. In collating the various chains, general themes emerge that describe classes of high-risk situations of which the offender must be wary and coping skill deficits that require remediation.

A variety of assessment techniques, in conjunction with the cognitive-behavioral chain of offense/relapse, will provide a relatively complete blueprint for treatment intervention. The preparation of an autobiography of the offender's life, a common assessment tool used in the treatment of sex offenders (Knopp, 1984), may be helpful in identifying familial and characterological factors that played a role in the offense. Similarly, the psychophysiological assessment of sexual arousal patterns through laboratory analogue techniques (Earls & Marshall, 1983; Laws & Osborn, 1983) can be employed to detect the role of deviant sexual arousal in the offense chain. Other factors such as social-skills deficits, substance abuse, impaired empathy towards others (particularly victims), sexual attitudes and dysfunctions, generally impaired impulse control and affect management, and low self-esteem can also be systematically assessed and related to the cognitive-behavioral chain.

HELPING THE OFFENDER PREVENT RELAPSE

As the offense chain is developed, the offender becomes more cognizant of the "danger signals" or "red flags" that foretell the impending risk for relapse. At each link in the chain, the offender explores interventions at the stimulus control level and the cognitive level. Stimulus control procedures, such as escape and avoidance, are emphasized to eliminate external stimuli (e.g., deviant pornography, being alone in the presence of a child, abusing alcohol or drugs, access to weapons). Each identified link or precursor is examined by the offender and therapist for alternative responses that reduce the risk of the situation and, consequently, decrease the chances of reoffense. Problem-solving techniques are applied so that a host of alternative coping responses can be generated, the list can be evaluated to determine whether each alternative would have the desired effect of minimizing the chances of reoffense, and the most effective alternative can be selected. Role plays and behavioral rehearsal assignments reinforce and enhance skill in the delivery of these alternative behaviors. In this fashion, more effective coping responses are programmed.

Identified AIDs are examined by the offender and therapist to expose their covert placement of the individual in a high-risk situation "unwittingly." The process of discovering the meaning and purpose of an AID robs it if value as a justification for the offense. Thus, the offender explores his "magical" or irrational thinking and develops a new mode of perception that focuses on the objective reality of the situation and moves the offender away from, rather than toward, the high-risk situation.

The further an offender progresses along a cognitive-behavioral chain culminating in a rape or molestation, the more difficult it is for him to intervene in a way that will prevent relapse. While it may be easier to correct an AID through appropriate self-talk than attempt to handle a lapse, it is often more difficult for the offender to recognize the AID. Therefore, the RP intervention requires a wide range of skill acquisitions and careful attention, on the part of both therapist and offender, to the range of choice points that the individual encounters in daily life. The offender must learn to identify those patterns that set the stage for a high-risk situation and be prepared to intervene at the earliest sign of the offense chain (Marques et al., 1984; Pithers et al., 1983).

Although a major focus of treatment from the RP perspective is teaching the offender to recognize and intervene early in the relapse chain, this approach also prepares the individual to handle the lapse and the associated AVE effectively, if and when it occurs. Central to this preparation is the emphasis that the offender remains at risk for reoffense even after a period of intensive treatment. Thus the notion of control as opposed to cure of the problem is reinforced. Because the lapse is predicted by the therapist, the offender can expect it and not be taken by surprise. An outline of steps for the offender to undertake to cope with the situation is prepared in advance. Though the plan must be individualized for each offender, it might include immediately engaging in specific activities that are incompatible with the lapse behavior; telephoning the therapist or other informed, supportive individual to assist in examining the lapse; giving self-instructions such as "the urge [to lapse] will dissipate whether I act on it or not"; and/or delaying the lapse for a certain specified time (e.g., twenty minutes). By contracting with the offender on this prepared plan of action for dealing with a lapse and rehearsing its execution, the offender enhances his sense of control, mastery, and self-efficacy (Marlatt, 1985; Marlatt & Gordon, 1980; Marques et al., 1984; Pithers et al., 1983).

One technique that can be used to cope with a lapse is the completion of a decision matrix. This technique requires the offender to consider the positive and negative consequences of reoffending and abstaining. It also forces the offender to focus on both the immediate and the delayed consequences of both behaviors. The matrix is a 2 (reoffend and abstain) × 2 (positive and negative) × 2 (immediate and delayed) table of consequences designed to remind the offender of the indulgent aspect of the sexually aggressive act, with its immediate gratification and delayed negative consequences

(Marlatt, 1985a; Marlatt & Gordon, 1980; Marques et al., 1984; Pithers et al., 1983). If it is unrealistic to expect the offender to complete a decision matrix at the time of a lapse, as it often is, a matrix can be prepared in advance and the offender can be instructed simply to refer to the matrix as part of the relapse contract.

Another technique that can be employed at the time of a lapse is for the offender to compare the positive effects he expects from engaging in the lapse with its actual effects (Marlatt, 1985b). For example, if the lapse is masturbation in response to a deviant fantasy, the offender may contract to list the positive effects he expects or hopes will accrue from the lapse behavior (e.g., sexual gratification, a sense of power or control). After the lapse, the offender would complete a similar list of the actual effects of committing the lapse (e.g., shame, guilt, challenging his sense of control and self-esteem). This technique can highlight the offender's unrealistic expectations for the deviant sexual behavior and propel him back toward a state of abstinence.

By preparing the offender for the occurrence of a lapse, the negative self-evaluation and dissonance of the accompanying AVE is reduced. Instead of interpreting the lapse as a sign of weakness, lack of willpower, and ineffective self-control, the offender can attribute it to a predictable part of the abstinence process. A self-statement such as "My therapist told me this is likely to occur, and now that it has I'm fortunate to have been prepared" can replace such relapse-engendering cognitions as "Treatment was ineffective, and I guess there is no way for me to control my sexual behavior." Also, the offender can be encouraged to construct and examine the cognitive-behavioral chain leading to the lapse in order to make it understandable and to construe it as a learning experience that can be positively used to avoid future lapses.

Treatment from an RP perspective is multimodal. Modalities that are commonly used in many sex offender treatment programs (Abel, Becker, & Skinner, 1985; Abel, Blanchard, & Becker, 1978; Annis, 1982; Freeman-Longo & Wells, 1986) are employed and integrated into a comprehensive system to assist the offender in decreasing the risk of relapse. A variety of behavioral techniques can be implemented to modify sexual arousal patterns (Quinsey & Marshall, 1983). Orgasmic reconditioning, for instance, can be employed to enhance sexual arousal in response to appropriate themes and objects (Foote & Laws, 1981; Kremsdorf, Holmen, & Laws, 1980; Laws & O'Neil, 1981; Marquis, 1970; VanDeventer & Laws, 1978). Conversely, olfactory aversion (Laws, Meyer, & Holmen, 1978; Maletzky, 1977), masturbatory satiation (Marshall, 1979; Marshall & Lippens, 1977), or covert sensitization (Davidson, 1968; Harbert, Barlow, Hersen, & Austin, 1974; Hayes, Brownell, & Barlow, 1978; Levin, Barry, Gamboro, Wolfinsohn, & Smith, 1977; Maletzky, 1980; Maletzky & George, 1973) can be used to decrease sexual arousal in response to undesirable themes or objects. Training to correct deficits in social, assertive, and empathic skills (Abel, 1976; Abel, Blanchard, & Becker, 1976, 1978; Peters, Pedigo, Steg, & McKenna, 1968; Peters & Roether, 1972) can also be implemented when indicated. Strategies directed at improving affect management—e.g., stress inoculation (Meichenbaum, 1977, 1985) and anger management therapy (Novaco, 1975)—can be employed for offenders who exhibit these problems. Substance abuse treatment (Donovan & Chaney, 1985; Marlatt & Gordon, 1980), when the problem is evident and serves as a disinhibitor of sexual aggression, can also be instituted. The RP model provides a way of integrating these various and diverse treatment interventions into a unified framework by referring back to the cognitive-behavioral chain of reoffense. This chain identifies high-risk elements and weaknesses in coping skills that can be targeted for modification, keeping both the offender and therapist oriented toward the rationale for employing the technique and its expected effect in aiding the control of relapse.

The offender described in the previously presented case illustration is presently engaged in treatment from an RP perspective. His behavior chains indicated that when confronted by a stressful interaction with his wife, his usual mode of coping (following his wife's direction) was ineffective. In fact, it was just that behavior which resulted in his negative feelings, because he perceived himself as a victim of her domination. This led him to spend more time in the presence of children, because in their presence he felt worthwhile and esteemed. When the offender was alone with a young girl during a period of unsatisfactory relations with his wife, he found himself becoming sexually aroused and he molested the child. An analysis of this chain of events indicated that the offender must learn to intervene at a number of levels on his behavior chain. Evaluation in the Sexual Behavior Laboratory confirmed the offender's self-report that he has a sexual preference for young girls. Therefore, olfactory aversion is being implemented to decrease his deviant arousal to pubescent females. Additionally, the offender's social skills deficit is reflected in his relationship with his wife, his difficulties on the job, and his lack of other appropriate adult relationships. The offender appeared to turn to children in times of stress partly because he did not have the requisite skills necessary to attract more appropriate friends. Treatment, therefore, also involves enhancing his affect management through stress inoculation and improving his social skills with adults. Finally, the offender's lack of empathy for his victims and his failure to completely come to grips with his own victimization allowed him to take the final step in the behavior chain and molest the child. Therefore, intervention aimed at having him examine the effects of his own sexual victimization has been implemented and is expected to enhance the offender's empathy for potential victims.

When exploring this case example, one can see that a diverse set of interventions is being applied. The structuring procedure is the behavior chain and its focus on AIDs, high-risk situations and the AVE. The offender learns to identify high-risk situations (i.e., being with children when no other adults are present) and their precursors. He learns to avoid them through the mastering of his newly acquired skills, or to escape the situation if avoidance is not possible. The offender also learns to identify the negative feelings associated with an AVE, and thus is not surprised and unable to cope with these feelings and the associated lapse.

CONCLUSIONS

Relapse Prevention, a self-control program designed to help people maintain behavioral changes by anticipating and coping with the problem of relapse, appears to be an appropriate model for intervention with sex offenders. The indulgent nature of rape or child molestation, with their short-term benefits followed by delayed negative consequences, allows one to compare reoffense with relapse to an addictive problem, such as alcoholism. The RP model provides a structure for the multimodal treatment of the sexual offender that defines reoffending as the result of a cognitive-behavioral chain.

Each link in this chain is a possible intervention point as the offender proceeds toward the offense through a series of choices (AIDs) which lead into high-risk situations. The offender's ability to cope with the different high-risk situations is the focus of treatment, as is the identification of the AIDs and the development of ways to avoid them. RP thus defines the goal of treatment as helping the offender to gain control over his behavior. It is grounded in developing a feeling of self-efficacy and effectiveness, not in offering a "cure" for deviant sexual behavior.

In this paper we have described the Relapse Prevention model and how it is being applied to sex offenders in one setting, the Sex Offender Treatment and Evaluation Project (SOTEP: Marques, 1985) at Atascadero State Hospital in California. While application of RP to a population such as ours appears appropriate and has been recommended previously (Marques et al., 1984; Pithers et al. 1983), it still awaits empirical confirmation. SOTEP is an experimental project designed to test the assumptions of the RP model with sexual aggressives and to explore the effectiveness of RP as a treatment model for incarcerated rapists and child molesters. Through implementation of the procedures described in this paper and an experimental design which includes longitudinal follow-up of matched, untreated controls, we expect to provide empirical evidence regarding the model's effectiveness with the population. SOTEP is presently in its third year of operation and has released 28 patients to aftercare.

NOTE

1. Because of the association of the acronym AIDs with Acquired Immune Deficiency Syndrome, a new acronym, SUBTLE (Seemingly Unimportant Behavior That Leads to Errors), has been proposed to designate the same process (Marlatt & Gordon, 1985, p. 49).

REFERENCES

Abel, G. G. (1976). Assessment of sexual deviation in the male. In M. Hersen & A. S. Bellack (Eds.), *Behavioral assessment: A practical handbook* (pp. 437-457). Elmsford, NY: Pergamon Press.

Abel, G. G., Becker, J. V., & Skinner, L. J. (1985). Behavioral approaches to treatment of the violent sex offender. In L. H. Roth (Ed.), *Clinical treatment of the violent person* (pp. 100-123) (DHHS Publication No. ADM 85-1425). Rockville, MD: National Institute of Mental Health.

Abel, G. G., Blanchard, E. B., & Becker, J. V. (1976). Psychological treatment of rapists. In M. J. Walker & S. L. Brodsky (Eds.), *Sexual assault: The victim and the rapist* (pp. 99-115). Lexington, MA: Lexington Books.

Abel, G. G., Blanchard, E. B., & Becker, J. V. (1978). An integrated treatment program for rapists. In R. Rada (Ed.), *Clinical aspects of the rapist* (pp. 161-214). New York: Grune & Stratton.

Abramson, L. Y., Seligman, M. E. P., & Teasdale, J. D. (1978). Learned helplessness in humans: Critique and reformulation. *Journal of Abnormal Psychology, 87*, 49-74.

Annis, L. V. (1982). A residential treatment program for male sex offenders. *International Journal of Offender Therapy and Comparative Criminology, 2*, 223-234.

Bandura, A. (1977). Self-efficacy: Toward a unifying theory of behavioral change. *Psychological Review, 84*, 191-215.

Brownell, K. D., Marlatt, G. A., Lichtenstein, E., & Wilson, G. T. (1986). Understanding and preventing relapse. *American Psychologist, 41*, 765-782.

Carnes, P. (1983). *The sexual addiction.* Minneapolis: Compcare.

Carnes, P. (1984). *Counseling the sexual addict.* Minneapolis: Compcare.

Davidson, G. (1968). Elimination of sadistic fantasy by a client-controlled counter-conditioning technique: A case study. *Journal of Abnormal Psychology, 73*, 84-90.

Donovan, D. M., & Chaney, E. F. (1985). Alcoholic relapse prevention and intervention: Models and methods. In G. A. Marlatt & J. R. Gordon (Eds.), *Relapse prevention: Maintenance strategies in the treatment of addictive behaviors* (pp. 351-416). New York: Guilford Press.

Earls, C. M., & Marshall, W. L. (1983). The current state of the technology in the laboratory assessment of sexual arousal patterns. In J. G. Greer & I. R. Stuart (Eds.), *The sexual aggressor: Current perspectives on treatment* (pp. 336-362). New York: Van Nostrand Reinhold.

Festinger, L. (1957). *A theory of cognitive dissonance.* Palo Alto, CA: Stanford University Press.

Foote, W. E., & Laws, D. R. (1981). A daily alternation procedure for orgasmic reconditioning with a pedophile. *Journal of Behavior Therapy and Experimental Psychiatry, 12*, 267-273.

Freeman-Longo, R., & Hall, R. V. (1986). Changing a lifetime of sexual crime. *Psychology Today, 20*(3), 58-64.

Harbert, T. L., Barlow, D. H., Hersen, M., & Austin, J. B. (1974). Measurement and modification of incestuous behavior: A case study. *Psychological Reports, 34*, 79-86.

Hayes, S. H., Brownell, K. D., & Barlow, D. H. (1978). The use of self-administered covert sensitization in the treatment of exhibitionism and sadism. *Behavior Therapy, 9*, 283-289.

Knopp, F. H. (1984). *Retraining adult sex offenders: Methods and models.* Syracuse, NY: Safer Society Press.

Kremsdorf, R. B., Holmen, M. L., & Laws, D. R. (1980). Orgasmic reconditioning without deviant imagery: A case report with a pedophile. *Behavior Research and Therapy, 18,* 203-207.

Laws, D. R., Meyer, J., & Holmen, M. L. (1978). Reduction of sadistic arousal by olfactory aversion: A case study. *Behavior Research and Therapy, 16,* 281-285.

Laws, D. R., & O'Neill, J. A. (1981). Variations on masturbatory conditioning. *Behavioral Psychotherapy, 9,* 111-136.

Laws, D. R., & Osborn, C. A. (1983). How to build and operate a behavioral laboratory to evaluate and treat sexual deviance. In J. G. Greer & I. R. Stuart (Eds.), *The sexual aggressor: Current perspectives on treatment* (pp. 293-335). New York: Van Nostrand Reinhold.

Maletzky, B. M. (1977). Booster sessions in aversion therapy: The permanency of treatment. *Behavioral Therapy, 8,* 460-463.

Marlatt, G. A. (1985a). Cognitive assessment and intervention procedures for relapse prevention. In G. A. Marlatt & J. R. Gordon (Eds.), *Relapse prevention: Maintenance strategies in the treatment of addictive behaviors* (pp. 128-200). New York: Guilford.

Marlatt, G. A. (1985b). Cognitive factors in the relapse process. In G. A. Marlatt & J. R. Gordon (Eds.), *Relapse prevention: Maintenance strategies in the treatment of addictive behaviors* (pp. 128-200). New York: Guilford.

Marlatt, G. A. (1985c). Relapse prevention: Theoretical rationale and overview of the model. In G. A. Marlatt & J. R. Gordon (Eds.), *Relapse prevention: Maintenance strategies in the treatment of addictive behaviors* (pp. 3-70). New York: Guilford.

Marlatt, G. A., & Gordon, J. R. (1980). Determinants of relapse: Implications for the maintenance of behavior change. In P. Davidson & S. Davidson (Eds.), *Behavioral medicine: Changing health lifestyles.* New York: Brunner/Mazel.

Marques, J. D. (1985). *Sex offender treatment and evaluation project: First report to the legislature in response to PC 1365.* Sacramento: California Department of Mental Health.

Marques, J. D., Pithers, W. D., & Marlatt, G. A. (1984). *Relapse prevention: A self-control program for sex offenders.* In California Department of Mental Health, *An innovative treatment program for sex offenders: Report to the legislature in response to 1983/84 Budget Act Item 4440-0110-001.* Sacramento: California Department of Mental Health.

Marquis, J. N. (1970). Orgasmic reconditioning: Changing sexual object choice through controlling masturbation fantasies. *Journal of Behavior Therapy and Experimental Psychiatry, 1,* 263-271.

Marshall, W. L. (1979). Satiation therapy: A procedure for reducing deviant arousal. *Journal of Applied Behavior Analysis, 12,* 377-389.

Marshall, W. L., & Lippens, K. (1977). The clinical value of boredom: A procedure for reducing inappropriate sexual interests. *Journal of Nervous and Mental Disease, 165,* 283-287.

Meichenbaum, D. (1977). *Cognitive-behavior modification.* New York: Plenum Press.

Meichenbaum, D. (1985). *Stress inoculation training.* New York: Pergamon Press.

Novaco, R. (1975). *Anger control: The development and evaluation of an experimental treatment.* Lexington, MA: D. C. Heath.

Peters, J., Pedigo, J., Steg, J., & McKenna, J. (1968). Group psychotherapy of the sex offender. *Federal Probation, 32,* 35-41.

Peters, J., & Roether, H. (1972). Group psychotherapy for probationed sex offenders. In H. L. Resnik & M. E. Wolfgang (Eds.), *Sexual behavior: Social, clinical and legal aspects* (pp. 255-266). Boston: Little, Brown.

Pithers, W. D., Marques, J. K., Gibat, C. C., & Marlatt, G. A. (1983). Relapse prevention with sexual aggressives: A self-control model of treatment and maintenance of change. In J. G. Greer & I. R. Stuart (Eds.), *The sexual aggressor: Current perspectives on treatment* (pp. 214-239). New York: Van Nostrand Reinhold.

Queen's Bench Foundation. (1976). *Rape: Prevention and resistance.* San Francisco, CA: Author.

Quinsey, V. L., & Marshall, W. L. (1983). Procedures for reducing inappropriate sexual arousal: An evaluation review. In J. G. Greer and I. R. Stuart (Eds.), *The sexual aggressor: Current perspectives on treatment* (pp. 267-289). New York: Van Nostrand Reinhold.

VanDeventer, A. D., & Laws, D. R. (1978). Orgasmic reconditioning to redirect sexual arousal in pedophiles. *Behavior Therapy, 9,* 748-765.

Issues in Treating Sex Offenders in the Community

John S. Wodarski
Daniel L. Whitaker

SUMMARY. Issues are presented that arise from the treatment of sex offenders in the community. Arguments are made regarding the need for serving this client population in the community as opposed to incarceration or hospitalization. Future research and treatment issues, as well as potential roadblocks to their resolution, are elaborated.

THE IMPACT OF LABELING ON TREATMENT

The public views the behavior of the labeled sex offender from a completely different perspective than for any other group of clients served in community mental health settings. This added labeling contributes to the difficulties of treating the sex offender who is identified with the nature of his crime on a negative, emotionally charged level. The general taboo of discussion in an open manner of sexual matters further hampers treatment. The attitude of the public is that the perpetrator deserves punishment for his "unmentionable" crimes. Consequently, the frequent assertion is that prison is the only suitable treatment context.

Due in part to the taboo nature of sex offenses, the general public, and professionals as well, often underestimate the number of persons seeking help for deviant sexual behavior. Many who exhibit behaviors falling under the rubric of sex offenses do not become involved in the formal judicial system. Moore, Zusman and Root (1985) report that almost one-half of the persons receiving treatment in the community mental health center were not "formally adjudicated" and that almost one-quarter had absolutely no contact with the criminal justice system. At times clients come to the community mental health center requesting help with unspecified distress. The sexual behavior is not revealed, or it is ignored, because it creates tension that is avoided by concentrating on less threatening therapeutic foci. The client is classified as seeking treatment for a psychiatric disorder not related to the sexual behavior and is not identified as a "sex offender." Such a therapeutic approach hampers requisite assessment and subsequent treatment planning.

Of course, if the person receives treatment without being labeled a sex offender, the lack of labeling may in itself be a positive event. As the sexual behavior has not been dealt with in a straightforward manner, however, the client often will become more confused and will view the mental health agency as unresponsive to his needs. If the client desires help in changing his sexual behavior, he feels frustrated and drops out of treatment. Dropping out is perceived as resistance to the "real" problem, that is the problem the agency perceives the client to have.

TREATABILITY

The prognosis for various sex offenders lies on a continuum, with repeat offenders who exhibit violent behaviors having the most negative prognosis. With adequate assessment and treatment, prognosis should surely increase (Overholser & Beck, 1986). Future research should address the psychological development of sexual offenders (Berlin & Meinecke, 1981; Berner, Brownstones, & Sluga, 1983; Cordoba & Chapel, 1983; Gagne, 1981). Moreover, the nature of other more general adjustment difficulties, e.g., interpersonal problems, need to be addressed (Fehrenbach, Smith, Monastersky, & Deisher, 1986; Margolin, 1984; Romero & Williams, 1983).

Many sexual behaviors result in extremely intense, pleasurable, and therefore highly reinforcing physiological changes. Certain types of sexual behavior are considered to be addictive for certain people (Carnes, 1983). Sexual behaviors have been found to be highly resistant to conventional treatment approaches and have at times been labeled incurable.

Data indicate that sexual offenders are not a homogeneous group of clients (Baxter, Marshall, Barbaree, Davidson, & Malcolm, 1984; Becker, Kaplan, Cuningham-Rathner, & Kavoussi, 1986; Erickson, Luxenberg, Walbek, & Seely, 1987; Malamuth, & Check, 1983; Quinsey, Chaplin, & Upfold, 1984). Some offenders, such as rapists, may need anger control, cognitive restructuring, social cues discrimination training, and so forth (Burgess, Jewitt, Sandham, & Hudson, 1980; Cohen, 1985; Lipton, McDonel, & McFall, 1987). Incest offenders need family therapy and interpersonal skills training. Thus more adequate conceptualization of the continuum of services is necessary. More theoretical development is necessary to account for the diversity of sexual offenders. Research needs to develop a taxonomy of treatable behaviors and related cost of adequate treatment. Stringent designs to isolate criteria for the provision of appropriate treatment interventions are a must. From the formulation of an adequate classification system would come the development of appropriate treatment paradigms.

The complexity of human sexual behavior is readily acknowledged. Yet our paradigms do not begin to capture this complexity. The future must produce more complex models of human behavior for utilization by social workers. These models most likely will be based on structural equation formulations and will incorporate such variables as biological predisposition, i.e., genes, electro-chemical imbalances and enzyme irregularities; cognitive variables; and the various social contexts with different rules of behavior interacting to produce changes (Wodarski, 1985).

Assessment of dangerousness is a very difficult clinical judgement to make. There are no known criteria which accurately discriminate the dangerous sex offender from the nondangerous sex offender (Aadland & Schag, 1984). Those criteria most often in use by clinicians are seldom seen as suitable by the public who believe that all sex offenders are dangerous and who therefore do not discriminate among types.

Legal decisions mandate that specific criteria must be developed for determining which offenders are dangerous, for determining who needs to be informed about potential dangerousness, and for isolating those offenders who can be treated in the community from those who need to be institutionalized (Alder, 1984; Nagayama·Hall

& Proctor, 1987; Naitove, 1985; Rada, 1978; Silver, 1976; Smith & Monastersky, 1986; Weiner, 1985). Such criteria will facilitate acceptance of those offenders who can be helped in the community with minimal risk, while high risk offenders are controlled. Labeling of all sex offenders as dangerous may eventually be reduced.

TREATMENT CONTEXT CONCERNS

For most sex offenses, there are victims of the act. With exhibitionists, for instance, there are often a number of persons who have been exposed to a most unpleasant experience. The victim feels uncomfortable and vulnerable. Many victims report a hypersensitivity which takes some time to subside. Where the offender is treated therefore becomes a major issue to the victim whose perception is frequently one of protection for the perpetrator and not for the victim.

At times, sex offenders are referred to a community mental health center for treatment as a result of a plea bargain agreement or as a condition of probation. Treatment at a community mental health center is not seen, and reasonably so, as punishment. If the perpetrator is simply released on condition of completion of a treatment program, victims do not believe their emotional damages have been properly compensated through adequate punishment of the perpetrator.

If the sex offense is incest, it is not unusual for the victim to be removed from the home while the perpetrator remains in the home. The child victim often perceives this as a punishment of her/him rather than of the perpetrator. At times it appears the family is more interested in perpetuating the family system than in considering the needs of the victim. Consequently, the victim receives threats and bribes from other members of the family system, including the perpetrator, to change his/her story.

There are many positive aspects in attempting to reach sex offenders while they remain in the community. If the perpetrator is placed on probation, it is possible for the family unit to reconcile and to remain intact as a family unit. If, on the other hand, he is absent from his family for a long period, the family tends to dissolve (Giarreto, 1982).

Care in the community generally is more efficient and helps insure the maintenance of achieved treatment goals. The environmental settings of prisons and hospitals are completely different from the community. Thus the behavioral changes which might take place as a result of counseling in these settings have little generalizability to the "real" world. Significant changes may be made, but because of the lack of opportunity to test these changes in vivo, they will not become a solid part of the prisoner's or patient's behavior repertoire. When experiencing the familiar negative affect or whatever antecedents led to the perpetrator's sexual behavior, the same familiar behavior patterns will emerge. The opportunity to practice alternative behaviors in the client's community and the preparation of significant others to support behavioral changes are essential. For example, the following are pertinent to the concepts of maintenance and generalization of behavior: training relatives or significant others in the client's environment, training behaviors that have a high probability of being reinforced in natural environments, varying the conditions of training, gradually removing or fading the contingencies, using different schedules of reinforcement, using delayed reinforcement and self control procedures, and so forth (Wodarski, 1987).

Unfortunately there are some drawbacks to community based treatment. Most community mental health centers and other public mental health treatment facilities are fairly open. Who receives treatment, and for what, frequently are common knowledge throughout the community. It is difficult to ensure confidentiality regarding the provision of services and even of what kind of group a particular client is attending. When the focus of treatment is on sexual problems, the opportunity for labeling increases. Provision of services to clients in the community also increases the probability of requests for testimony on client behavior.

A number of conflicts arise from the delivery of treatment to sexual offenders in community settings. Many community mental health facilities are mandated to provide mental health services to all regardless of ability to pay. This means that at times agencies will provide services to both the sex offender and to his/her victim. This can create the appearance of a conflict of interest. It may appear to the victim that, as the perpetrator is receiving equal services, their fears and concerns are not being adequately addressed (Moore, Zusman, & Root, 1985).

Finally, if a community mental health center provides services for sex offenders, a certain notoriety is attached to the center. Such notoriety can make it more difficult for the center to properly serve other clients who may avoid the center unless there is no alternative. Again, public education is needed to reduce these fears.

COST OF TREATMENT

Another critical issue, which incidentally is related to that of generalization and maintenance of behavior, is the cost of therapy. Generalization and maintenance procedures incorporated into treatment programs increase initial costs but are cost effective in the long run. The cost of hospitalization in mental hospitals is extremely high. Certain estimates are in excess of $380/day. Likewise, the estimates of incarceration are high. In certain instances, the cost of maintaining, without treatment, a sex offender in a prison-type setting exceeds $20,000/year. The cost of treatment in a noninstitutional setting, on the other hand, can be less than $500/ month. Not only does it cost less to provide services on a community basis because of prisoner or patient capital costs, it also is less costly because there is the opportunity for the perpetrator to provide for his/her family's care.

In terms of human costs, community treatment furthermore is indicated. In the community incest perpetrators retain the opportunity to modify family relationships and to establish a supportive, as opposed to an exploitive, relationship. The process of treatment would be one of acceptance of responsibility, establishment or reestablishment of the marital and parent-child dyads, and then reconstitution of the family as a supportive environment. The family is not torn asunder and made dependent on the welfare system but remains intact and solvent.

Social decency offenders likewise may retain family responsibilities as they participate in treatment. The emotional support from their families would substantially improve the probability of success in treatment. It would moreover provide a source of immediate feedback as to progress in making improvements in interpersonal relationships.

PREVENTION AND TREATMENT

All sex offender treatment programs should include a prevention component. One aspect of that component should be an emphasis on the discussion of sexual deviance in a forthright, nonjudgmental manner. The inability to discuss sexual matters without an increase in tension continues to make it difficult to provide services to sex offenders.

The development of different typologies of sex offenders and the derivation of relevant treatment strategies are currently in the pilot stage of development. Research is needed to determine the potential for sexual offenses. More instruments such as the Rape Index that specifies the potential for rape and matches client assessments with relevant treatment need to be developed (Davidson & Malcolm, 1985).

At the current stage of development, it would be best to go with comprehensive broad-based treatment packages and subsequently to delineate the relevancy of each aspect of the package. Much accumulated research seems to indicate that a life skills approach based on knowledge about sexuality, cognitive restructuring, problem solving, interpersonal skills, and anger management is preferable (Becker, 1978). Critical components of treatment packages cannot be isolated through single-subject designs, which serve mainly to isolate those packages that need refinement. The only designs capable of isolating critical components are factorial designs with adequate controls. Complex designs will provide answers to the relevant practice questions of who, where, when, how long, and with what intervention.

THE ADOLESCENT OFFENDER

A significant challenge to the field is the provision of services for the adolescent sex offender. According to Davis and Leitenberg (1987), recent arrest statistics and surveys indicate that:

about 20% of all rapes and about 30% to 50% of all cases of child sexual abuse can be attributed to adolescent offenders (Brown, Flanagan, & McLeod, 1984; Deisher, Wenet, Paperny, Clark, & Fehrenbach, 1982). In addition, approximately 50% of adult sex offenders report that their first sexual offense occurred during adolescence (Abel, Mittelman, & Becker, 1985; Becker & Abel, 1985; Gebhard, Gagnon, Pomeroy, & Christenson, 1965; Groth, Longo, & McFadin, 1982; Smith, 1984). Although this does not mean that 50% of adolescent sex offenders continue committing sexual offenses into adulthood, enough obviously do to warrant serious concern. (p. 417)

CONCLUSION

The treatment of certain sex offenders in the community makes sense in terms of social and monetary costs. Individuals will be less demoralized while more family units will be preserved. The community will become more supportive through education and adequate provision of treatment for the offenders and their victims. The development and provision of appropriate services, however, represent a substantial challenge. The necessary research to accomplish these goals has yet to be undertaken.

We must first take a look at the composition of services in our social system. The provision of services in institutions where individuals labeled as deviant are served along with others so labeled has significant drawbacks. According to Bandura's social modeling theory, this process facilitates the modeling of deviant behaviors. It may be that modification of behavior is best accomplished through structuring differently the delivery of the services. When sex offenders are treated in the community, the community does not have to provide the direct costs of maintenance of the perpetrator in a hospital or prison, nor does it have to provide welfare costs for the dependent family. In addition, most sex offenders could, if not prevented by incarceration, make significant contributions to society. However, research has yet to isolate the number of sex offenders who are not motivated to secure appropriate community treatment (Fein & Bishop, 1987).

It must be determined why sexually deviant behaviors are so resistant to change. The progressive approach of Marlatt and Gordon (1985) that calls for applying with sexual aggressives the relapse prevention model developed for use in the treatment of addictive behaviors is an example of the type of applied research that will address the critical issue of treatability. Once treated, we need to recognize and apply the various procedures that can be readily employed for the maintenance of achieved behavioral changes. Cost effectiveness of both treatment and maintenance strategies remains a major concern.

Many therapists have objected to serving sex offenders. They feel inadequately trained, or because of their own personal histories and personal bias, they do not believe that they can adequately treat sex offenders. It is certainly important that personnel working with sex offenders be capable of accepting the sex offender as a person. Educational issues in the preparation of practitioners therefore need to be addressed.

Finally, public education programs are needed to inform the public regarding which individuals can be treated in the community with the least risk. Only through education will the misconceptions and public roadblocks that hamper treatment of the sexual offender be removed.

REFERENCES

Aadland, R. L., & Schag, D. S. (1984). The assessment of continued threat to the community in a mentally ill offender program. *Journal of Criminal Justice, 12*, 81-86.

Abel, G. G., Mittelman, M. S., & Becker, J. V. (1985). Sexual offenders: Results of assessment and recommendations for treatment. In H. H. Ben-Aron, S. I. Hucker, & C. D. Webster (Eds.), *Clinical criminology* (pp. 191-205). Toronto, Ontario, Canada: MM Graphics.

Alder, C. (1984). The convicted rapist: A sexual or a violent offender? *Criminal Justice and Behavior, 11*(2), 157-177.

Baxter, D. J., Marshall, W. L., Barbaree, H. E., Davidson, P. R., & Malcolm, P. B. (1984). Deviant sexual behavior: Differentiating sex offenders by criminal and personal history, psychometric measures, and sexual response. *Criminal Justice and Behavior, 11*(4), 477-501.

Becker, J. V. et al. (1978). Evaluating social skills of sexual aggressives. *Criminal Justice & Behavior, 5*(4), 357-368.

Becker, J. V., & Abel, G. G. (1985). *Methodological and ethical issues in evaluating and treating adolescent sexual offenders* (Pub. No. ADM-85-1396). Rockville, MD: U.S. Department of Health and Human Services.

Becker, J. V., Kaplan, M. S., Cunningham-Rathner, J., & Kavoussi, R. (1986). Characteristics of adolescent incest sexual perpetrators: Preliminary findings. *Journal of Family Violence, 1*(1), 85-97.

Berlin, F. S., & Meinecke, C. F. (1981). Treatment of sex offenders with antiandrogenic medication: Conceptualization, review of treatment modalities, and preliminary findings. *American Journal of Psychiatry, 138*(5), 601-607.

Berner, W., Brownstone, G., & Sluga, W. (1983). The cyproteronacetat treatment of sexual offenders. *Neuroscience & Biobehavioral Reviews, 7*(3), 441-443.

Brown, E. J., Flanagan, T. J., & McLeod, M. (Eds.). (1984). *Sourcebook of criminal justice statistics – 1983*. Washington, DC: Bureau of Justice Statistics.

Burgess, R., Jewitt, R., Sandham, J., & Hudson, B. L. (1980). Working with sex offenders: A social skills training group. *British Journal of Social Work, 10*, 133-142.

Carnes, P. J. (1983). *Sexual addiction*. Minneapolis, MN: CompCare Press.

Cohen, B. Z. (1985). A cognitive approach to the treatment of offenders. *British Journal of Social Work, 15*, 619-633.

Cordoba, O. A., & Chapel, J. L. (1983). Medroxyprogesterone acetate antiandrogen treatment of hypersexuality in a pedophiliac sex offender. *American Journal of Psychiatry, 140*(8), 1036-1039.

Davidson, P. R., & Malcolm, P. B. (1985). The reliability of the rape index: A rapist sample. *Behavioral Assessment, 7*, 283-292.

Davis, G. E., & Leitenberg, H. (1987). Adolescent sex offenders. *Psychological Bulletin, 101*(3), 417-427.

Deisher, R. W., Wenet, G. A., Paperny, D. M., Clark, T. F., & Fehrenbach, P. A. (1982). Adolescent sexual offense behavior: The role of the physician. *Journal of Adolescent Health Care, 2*, 279-286.

Erickson, W. D., Luxenberg, M. G., Walbek, N. H., & Seely, R. K. (1987). Frequency of MMPI two-point code types among sex offenders. *Journal of Consulting and Clinical Psychology, 55*(4), 566-570.

Fehrenbach, P. A., Smith, W., Monastersky, C., & Deisher, R. W. (1986). Adolescent sexual offenders: Offender and offense characteristics. *American Journal of Orthopsychiatry, 56*(2), 225-233.

Fein, E., & Bishop, G. V. (1987). Child sexual abuse: Treatment for the offender. *Social Casework, 68*(2), 122-124.

Gagne, P. (1981). Treatment of sex offenders with medroxyprogesterone acetate. *American Journal of Psychiatry, 138*(5), 644-646.

Gebhard, P. H., Gagnon, J. H., Pomeroy, W. B., & Christenson, C. V. (1965). *Sex offenders: An analysis of types*. New York: Harper & Row.

Giarretto, H. (1982). *Integrated treatment of child sexual abuse: A treatment and training manual*. Palo Alto, CA: Science and Behavior Books.

Groth, A. N., Longo, R. E., & McFadin, J. B. (1982). Undetected recidivism among rapists and child molesters. *Crime and Delinquency, 28,* 450-458.

Lipton, D. N., McDonel, E. C., & McFall, R. M. (1987). Heterosocial perception in rapists. *Journal of Consulting and Clinical Psychology, 55*(1), 17-21.

Malamuth, N. M., & Check, J. V. P. (1983). Sexual arousal to rape depictions: Individual differences. *Journal of Abnormal Psychology, 92*(1), 55-67.

Margolin, L. (1984). Group therapy as a means of learning about the sexually assaultive adolescent. *International Journal of Offender Therapy & Comparative Criminology, 28*(1), 65-72.

Marlatt, G. A., & Gordon, J. R. (1985). *Relapse prevention: Maintenance strategies in the treatment of addictive behaviors.* New York: Guilford.

Moore, H. A., Zusman, J., & Root, G. C. (1985). Noninstitutional treatment for sex offenders in Florida. *American Journal of Psychiatry, 142*(8), 964-967.

Nagayama Hall, G. C., & Proctor, W. C. (1987). Criminological predictors of recidivism in a sexual offender population. *Journal of Consulting and Clinical Psychology, 55*(1), 111-112.

Naitove, C. E. (1985). Protecting our children: The fight against molestation. *The Arts in Psychotherapy, 12,* 115-116.

Overholser, J. C., & Beck, S. (1986). Multimethod assessment of rapists, child molesters, and three control groups on behavioral and psychological measures. *Journal of Consulting and Clinical Psychology, 54*(5), 682-687.

Quinsey, V. L., Chaplin, T. C., & Upfold, D. (1984). Sexual arousal to nonsexual violence and sadomasochistic themes Among rapists and non-sex-offenders. *Journal of Consulting and Clinical Psychology, 52*(4), 651-657.

Rada, R. T. (1978). Legal aspects in treating rapists. *Criminal Justice & Behavior, 5*(4), 369-378.

Romero, J. J., & Williams, L. M. (1983). Group psychotherapy and intensive probation supervision with sex offenders: A comparative study. *Federal Probation, 47*(4), 36-42.

Silver, S. N. (1976). Outpatient treatment for sexual offenders. *Social Work, 21*(2), 134-140.

Smith, W. R. (1984). Patterns of re-offending among juvenile sexual offenders. Unpublished manuscript, University of Washington, Juvenile Sexual Offender Program, Seattle.

Smith, W. R., & Monastersky, C. (1986). Assessing juvenile sex offenders' risk for re-offending. *Criminal Justice and Behavior, 13,* 115-140.

Weiner, B. A. (1985). Legal issues raised in treating sex offenders. *Behavioral Sciences & the Law, 3*(4), 325-340.

Wodarski, J. S. (1985). *Introduction to human behavior.* Austin, TX: PRO-ED.

Wodarski, J. S. (1987). *Social work practice with children and adolescents.* Springfield, IL: Charles C Thomas.

Index

Induced dream technique. *See*
Hypnotherapy
Intervention
for abuse victims, 110
for mentally retarded sex offenders, 41,
42,44,46
for rapists and child molesters, 139
for sexually aggressive youth, 4,95,103,
105

J

Juvenile Sexual Offender Program
(University of Washington
Hospital), 95

K

Kinsey Sex Institute, 51

L

Labeling of sex offenders
impact on treatment, 145-46,148,149
Lapse, 132,133,136,137,139
versus relapse, 131

M

Maintenance strategies, 150,153
Masochists, 20
Masturbation, 10,22,38,40,49,138
criminal in some jurisdictions, 55-56
Masturbatory satiation, 92
Mental retardation
relation to sexual delinquency, 36,38,
39-41,43,45-46
Mentally disordered sex offender (MDSO)
laws
controversy over, 53
Mentally retarded persons
delayed sexual development, 40
inconclusive evidence of sexual
deviancy, 38-41,45
lack of sexual knowledge, 40,44
sex drive, 35,40,45

sexual rights controversy, 34-35,45
Mentally retarded sex offenders
lack of research concerning, 43
risks of research, 45
treatment for, 41-43,44-45,46
Minnesota Multiphasic Personality
Inventory (MMPI) profiles, 51-52,
59,62
Modeling
of deviant behaviors, 152
Molestation
defined, 2,36
death-penalty demanded, 50
Mothers
of sex offenders, 56

N

New Jersey Diagnostic Center, 51

O

Oregon State Hospital, Social Skills Unit of
Correctional Treatment Program, 42

P

Paraphilia, 3,20
Parents United, 73
Pedophiles
aversion therapy, 13
drug therapy, 20
high fantasy activity, 6
hypnosis treatment, 6-7
Pharmacotherapy, 19-22
antiandrogen drug therapy, 20,21,24
Preadolescent sexual offenders, 89,91,
96-97,99-100,102,104-5,107,111-12
Premarital sex, 49
Prevention
emphasis on, 151
Prevention of sex offenses, 63,65
Probation of sex offenders, 1
success of, 5
Psychodynamic therapy
in treatment of sex offenders, 5,7-9
Psychotherapy, fantasy-oriented